Memory and nerve cell connections

Memory and nerve cell connections

CRITICISMS AND CONTRIBUTIONS FROM DEVELOPMENTAL NEUROPHYSIOLOGY

BY

RICHARD MARK

PHYSIOLOGY DEPARTMENT
MONASH UNIVERSITY

CLARENDON PRESS · OXFORD

Oxford University Press, Ely House, London W.1

GLASGOW NEW YORK TORONTO MELBOURNE WELLINGTON
CAPE TOWN IBADAN NAIROBI DAR ES SALAAM LUSAKA ADDIS ABABA
DELHI BOMBAY CALCUTTA MADRAS KARACHI DACCA
KUALA LUMPUR SINGAPORE HONG KONG TOKYO

Casebound ISBN 0 19 857126 7
Paperback ISBN 0 19 857129 1

© OXFORD UNIVERSITY PRESS 1974

First published in 1974
Reprinted 1975

PRINTED IN GREAT BRITAIN BY
FLETCHER AND SON LTD
NORWICH

TO

Gerda, Bettina and David,
real trees, in the forests of
imagination.

The brain is so imperfectly understood that we simply do not know enough about its physiology and function to deduce facts about its performance.

GERMAINE GREER, *The female eunuch* (1970).

Preface

THE physiological approach to memory is to try to discover the mechanism. This resides in the brain, an organ of overwhelming complexity. How can one think about a mechanism of memory, when the way in which the brain controls the simplest of behaviour is still mysterious, and when the topic of memory comes so close to the still unformulated problems of the relation of the brain to conscious experience and personal identity? One strategy is to select an aspect of the mechanism that has the most in common with other biological knowledge and on which current scientific and technical advances can be brought to bear. In this way real progress in understanding can be made, providing both insight and methods for the next exploratory steps. Like other tissues of the body, all brains are composed of cells, and sooner or later, in some way, events to be remembered must make a lasting change in the way brain cells work. There must be some biochemical switch which is indispensable for the storage of memory. If one knows about the physiology of nerve cells it is not too difficult to make testable predictions as to what kind of process might be needed.

This book is intended as a guide, a short argument in favour of one of these predictions about the cellular nature of memory, which has emerged from developments in the last ten years in research on the biochemistry, physiology, and embryology of the vertebrate brain. It does not review all the immense literature of memory in an objective fashion. Marie Gibbs and I have attempted some of this elsewhere (1973). The job of a guide, is to take you through a territory with which he is thoroughly familiar and where it may be dangerous to go alone, and to provide a viewpoint from which some special features may be enjoyed. What you then make of them is your own affair. You may be pleasantly surprised by what you see, or you may be disappointed; in which case you will certainly choose a different guide next time.

These ideas began to develop in the few years I spent in Professor R. W. Sperry's laboratory at the California Institute of Technology. I am also aware of the influence of other members of the Biology Division there, specially Max Delbruck and Seymour Benzer. I thank Brian Cragg and Professors J. Z. Young and G. A. Horridge for their interest, help, and encouragement, and I look back with pleasure to laboratory work done in Professor A. K. McIntyre's department at Monash University with Lauren Marotte and Marie Gibbs (Watts).

I am grateful for support from the Australian Research Grants Committee. I thank Diana Harrison for the illustrations, Barbara Genat for assistance with the bibliography and manuscript, and Lynne Hepburn for preparing the final draft.

Contents

1 *Neurophysiology*

NERVE CELLS

THE cellular components of the brains of all animals are remarkably similar (Horridge, 1968). The functions of co-ordinating movement of the animal, of receiving impressions of the outside world, and acting on the impressions received, are handled by a collection of specialized cells mainly of ecto-dermal origin. Primitive invertebrates show instances where the epithelial tissue covering the animal develops patches or strips that appear to be able to co-ordinate the function of attached cilia and of muscles beneath. In the more complex animals specialized ectoderm becomes separate from the epithelial covering and is buried in the mesoglea or mesoderm. Cell extensions reach to other sensory cells on the surface, and to strings of muscle cell below. Disturbances on the surface of the animal are signalled by the primitive nerve cells to produce co-ordinated contractions of the muscular coat (Fig. 1).

Many of the nerve cells in the simplest of metazoa show evidence of intercellular communication by secretory activity, which is characteristic of nervous tissue everywhere. In fact the similiarity in origin, structure, and function of nervous tissue in all motile animals yet examined would suggest that, for this evolutionary problem of the rapid distribution of in-formation between cells, only one solution has come to be relied upon, just as the nucleic acids appear to be universally used to carry information between generations. The specializa-tions of nerve cells, or neurones, are basically similar in all

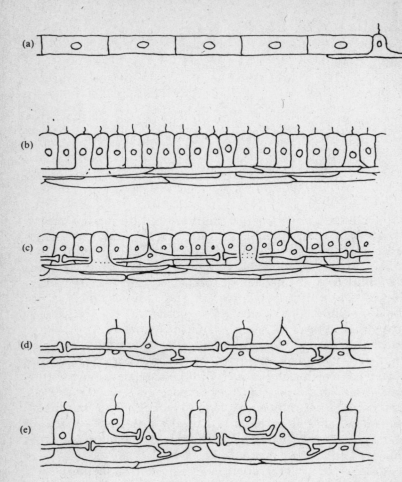

FIG. 1. The origin of the nerve cell. (*a*) Conducting epithelium leading to an epithelial muscle cell. (*b*) Muscle cells connected by their tails. (*c*) As in (*b*), but with epithelial cells with processes that connect only with each other and bridge over intervening cells. This is the critical stage of appearance of axons, and there is no clue as to which type of cell gave rise to them. (*d*) Connections to muscle cells. (*e*) Origin of sensory cells, after the appearance of conducting systems. (After Horridge, 1968.)

animals, vertebrates and invertebrates, and in all parts of the nervous system. There are important sub-specializations among neurones, but the fundamental capabilities of nerve cells are invariant. Just as genetics can be studied in creatures from viruses to man, so neurophysiology and neurobiology can draw from observations on the nervous system of any animal. This gives a unity to the study of the brain, even to the highest functions of human perception and memory, that can greatly accelerate the growth of understanding. Experiments on neurones that are accessible to study can suggest whether or not certain properties might account for the behaviour of parts of the brain where, for technical reasons, the same experiments are not possible, either because of the minute size of the cells, or the complexity of their arrangement.

Electrical signalling

The most obvious specialization of some nerve cells that function as units of a brain is an enormous increase in length, coupled with the elaboration of a property, common to the membranes of some other cells in plants and animals, of propagating a temporary disturbance set up in one part of the cell until it traverses the whole membrane. The nature of this disturbance in nerve cells is a transient electrochemical change in the membrane, which spreads rapidly, and can be detected as a wave which cancels and momentarily reverses the small (50–70 mV) potential difference between the inside and outside of one cell.

The signals generated by nerve cells are well within the range of sensitivity of present-day electronic instruments. For faithful recording of the action potential, an intracellular electrode must be made fine enough to penetrate the cell membrane, and remain inside without significant damage. Glass pipettes filled with a conducting solution, and with tips less than 0·2 μm in diameter, are usually used, and this enables the potential difference across the membrane to be measured directly. Because the changes with an action potential are so fast, the measuring instrument is usually a cathode-ray oscilloscope, in which a beam of electrons sweeping over a phosphorescent screen at a constant speed, is deflected by the amplified nervous signal, to produce a graph of potential change versus time.

The physical change in the membrane that accompanies this wave is not yet understood, but it is known to produce rapid sequential alterations in the permeability of the membrane to some of the smaller ions found inside and outside the

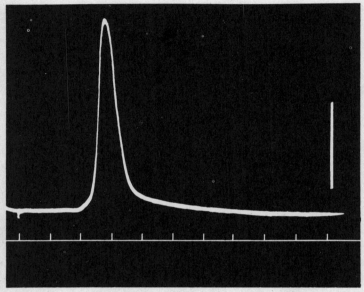

FIG. 2. The universal signal. An action potential recorded by a micro-electrode inside a nerve cell of the cat spinal cord. The resting potential of the cell was −70 mV momentarily reversed and returned to normal. Time scale, ms; voltage 50 mV. (After McIntyre, Mark, and Steiner, 1956.)

cells. The potential wave is carried by the ionic currents that are allowed to flow in and out for very brief periods. In most cells the depolarizing wave is carried mainly by a flow of Na+ current into the cell, and the repolarization of the membrane at the end of the transient change is produced by K+ current flowing out. Both changes may be over in a few milliseconds (Fig. 2).

The wave of potential change, known as the action potential or spike potential because it is so brief, propagates by local current flow between active and resting membrane. An active area of the membrane that has lost or reversed its membrane potential, induces current to flow through neighbouring inactive areas. This current flow passively lowers the membrane potential until a critical level is reached, upon which ionic permeabilities suddenly change, and the membrane potential collapses and may momentarily reverse.

The sequence of permeability changes is triggered by a membrane mechanism that is voltage dependent, and the exact threshold can change in a number of ways. Once begun, however, the changes appear to be more or less invariant and always result in an all-or-nothing permeability change of constant magnitude and timing. This signal sweeps over the whole cell, travelling in some large diameter nerve fibres at a velocity of 100 m s, and slower in smaller fibres.

Differences in ionic concentration between the inside and outside of the cell, a universal feature of living cells, are maintained by ion pumps working continuously against the concentration gradients they build up. The membrane is kept charged by chemical reactions powered from the metabolism of the cell. The ionic imbalance resulting from the passage of the action potential is very small compared with the total amounts of intracellular ions, and the exact ion concentrations are restored by the continued activity of the ion pumps. A nerve fibre can carry many successive action potentials with little or no expenditure of metabolic energy. The recovery process after thousands of impulses can, however, be very long, of the order of minutes, whereas each action potential takes only milliseconds (Hodgkin, 1964).

Nerve cells in the brain

The increase in cell length, which may go as far as increasing the ratio between cell diameter and cell length to 1 000 000 : 1, produces conducting pathways over which any disturbance set up at one end will propagate unchanged to the other end. It becomes a single transmission line, which will reproduce at one end any signal applied at the other end, with no loss of signal but with a certain time delay. The brain of man contains some 10^{12} of these units, or neurones, of many different shapes and sizes, packed within a 1200-ml space. Most neuronal cell bodies containing the nucleus are in or very near

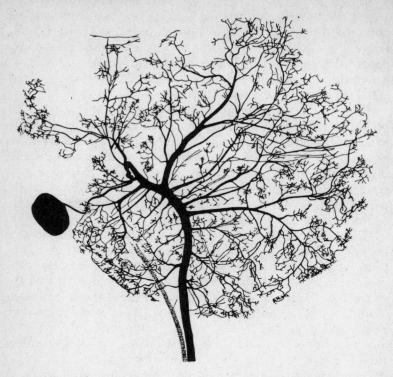

FIG. 3. A nerve cell. This one, from the Australian plague locust, *Chortoicetes*, has been outlined in its entirety by injection with cobalt ions which are subsequently precipitated as the black sulphide. The nucleus is in the ovoid expansion to the left and the axon, which is destined to form contacts with a muscle cell, continues on from the thickened shaft at the bottom. Terminals from other nerve cells end all over the branching dendritic tree. They are not stained by this method and can only be clearly seen by the electronmicroscope. (From Dr. Mark Tyer.)

the brain or spinal cord. Their thin and branching processes mostly remain within the central nervous system, but some extend out into other parts of the body in bundles, usually of many thousands of fibres together; these are the peripheral nerves to skin, muscle, and internal organs (Fig. 3). This specialization of nerve cells to single signal transmission units is particularly remarkable in that it also holds under conditions of very close packing in the brain, and also in spite of enormous variations in cell geometry. The reason for the ability of nerve cells to transmit a membrane disturbance or impulse along themselves, without significantly influencing their neighbours, is found in another special feature of brain anatomy, again occurring almost without exception through the species. Unlike cells of some other tissues, neurones are not packed tightly together to form solid sheets or masses. Surrounding each nerve cell is a narrow gap, in some cases only 200 A wide, which separates each cell from the others in the brain. This gap is normally filled with tissue fluid and certain macromolecules, and appears to be of crucial importance to the function of the brain. It provides the low-resistance electrical pathway through which any electrical disturbance, propagated as an action potential in one cell, will flow. It acts to short-circuit current flows which might otherwise have penetrated adjacent cell membranes, and tended to set up unwanted electrical disturbances which could then begin to propagate as nerve impulses. The biochemical control of the width of this gap is not well understood, although it is recognized as an important problem in brain research (Van Harreveld, 1966).

A fine glass or wire electrode may be placed outside a nerve cell in the extracellular fluid phase of the brain, and a sensitive electronic system used to measure the potential difference between this and a remote electrode. The extracellular current flow round a nerve cell induces a potential difference between an electrode very close to the membrane, and one far away. If the electrode is small and well placed it may record the activity of only one cell, in which case the method is called extracellular unit recording. This has been a most useful method in the modern physiology of the central nervous system. If the electrode is large in comparison with the dimensions of nerve cells, its potential will be influenced by hundreds or thousands of adjacent nerve cells, although the contribution of each one to the potential change is now much smaller. If the contributing nerve cells are discharging asynchronously their potential contributions will tend to cancel out. If by artificial, electrical, or other stimulation, they are made to fire impulses all together then the size of the resultant evoked potential will give some measure of the number of neurones contributing. This method has also been used extensively in mapping out the central nervous system.

FUNCTIONAL CONNECTIONS BETWEEN NERVE CELLS

Linkage of nerve cell units into the functional network of the brain requires a specific, organized breakdown of this effective barrier between cells so that activity in one cell can be transferred to certain neighbouring units while remaining isolated from all others. There are two ways in which this is brought about. In certain brain systems, once again found in both vertebrates and invertebrates, the gap between certain cells is closed, the cell membranes grow together, and then undergo a change in structure which reduces the transverse membrane resistance. Quite similar junctions between cells are found in other tissues, notably heart cells. In the brain, the effect on the impulse-carrying mechanisms of nerve cells is to link two cells electrically, so that the propagated impulse once started in one cell will sweep over both cell membranes as if they were one. These electrical connections between cells do not form in a haphazard manner, and do not work without the specific morphological changes in the cell membranes at their site of opposition. This method of connecting nerve cells is not common in the brain. Two cells linked in such a manner normally behave as one, as far as impulse pattern is concerned, and it is apparent that a system connected up entirely by these junctions would not have particularly interesting or powerful properties of information handling. It does provide a reliable connection between nerve cells, and ensures that the synchronization of activity patterns of the two cells is accomplished with the minimum of time delay. In certain circumstances this is important in the evolution of nervous control.

Excitatory chemical synapses

The majority of intercellular connections in the brain are made through a more complicated structure, the synapse or synaptic junction. There is little direct electrical linkage between cells. The extracellular gap remains, and it is still an effective insulator of impulse activity.

Information is carried between the neurones by a localized, pulse-like, secretion, into the intercellular gap of a substance which will change the electrical properties of a patch of the membrane of the adjacent cell. The change alters the permeability of the membrane to ions in solution, both inside and outside the cell membrane, in a similar way to the change causing the action potential. It differs slightly in that it is chemically induced by the transmitter substance, not by the internal voltage-dependent membrane mechanism of the action potential. The permeability change is less selective than in the case of the action potential, and results in a very brief collapse of membrane potential over the chemically sensitive area. The current pulse thus injected into the membrane induces a slower attenuated current flow in adjacent areas of membrane. The resulting depolarization and gradual repolarization of the cell membrane potential can be recorded by an electrode placed within the cell. It is called an excitatory postsynaptic potential, or e.p.s.p. If this is strong enough to depolarize adjacent membrane to the threshold level, the action potential mechanism is activated. Once this happens, the impulse travels over the new cell, carried by the action-potential mechanism, and the process of synaptic transmission may be repeated at other synaptic junctions, or until the impulse leaves the central nervous system down nerve fibres to muscle or gland cells where an exactly similar process of secretory transmission of the nerve impulse can trigger glandular secretion or the contraction of a muscle fibre.

Synapses, which are presumed to act by secretion of a transmitter substance, will normally only transmit in one direction. The cytochemical specialization underlying this is shown by electronmicrographic studies which reveal a different appearance of pre-synaptic elements and post-synaptic elements. Pre-synaptic endings of nerve cells, from which the transmitter substance is presumed to be released, contain a dense-packed collection of small vesicles almost 500 A in diameter in close apposition to the membrane of the synapse. It has been suggested that the vesicles actually contain the transmitter substance and participate in the mechanism of its release, although proof of this very reasonable assertion is difficult to obtain. The post-synaptic cell does not normally contain vesicles and presumably therefore can release no transmitter into the synaptic cleft between the extracellular membranes (Fig. 4) (Katz, 1969).

From this polarization of synaptic structure it follows that conduction of information over a nerve cell under normal conditions is always in one direction. By convention cell branches which conduct towards the cell body are called dendrites, and the branches which conduct away from the cell body are called axons. There is usually only one main axon for each cell which may break up into a terminal bush at its distal end. Although the whole of the cell, dendrites, cell body, and axon, may act as post-synaptic elements in nervous networks, most commonly only the axon and the terminal axon branches act as pre-synaptic elements. There are, however, occasional descriptions of cell-to-cell contacts particularly in the thalamus and olfactory organs of animals in which it appears that both elements involved and dendritic.

Effectiveness of excitatory synaptic transmission

In some synapses, particularly those on pathways leading from sense organs to the central nervous system, the efficiency of transmission may be extremely high. In synaptic junctions of the spinal cord concerned with relaying information from skin and joint receptors to the cerebral cortex, one isolated impulse set up in a single fibre of a peripheral sensory nerve may penetrate at least two synaptic relays to generate a response at the cerebral cortex. Morphological study of one of these synapses shows several features which may account for this efficiency of transmission. The pre-synaptic terminals are extremely large compared to other synaptic junctions and form bulbous expansions along the length of terminal segments of the axon, which are applied at intervals along the length of the elongated cell body of the post-synaptic cell. Increase in the area of synaptic contact means that there is a relatively large area of post-synaptic membrane on which the secretory product of the pre-synaptic element may act. A large area of post-synaptic membrane will be activated almost at one moment and the probability of the development of a propagated action potential in the post-synaptic cell greatly increased.

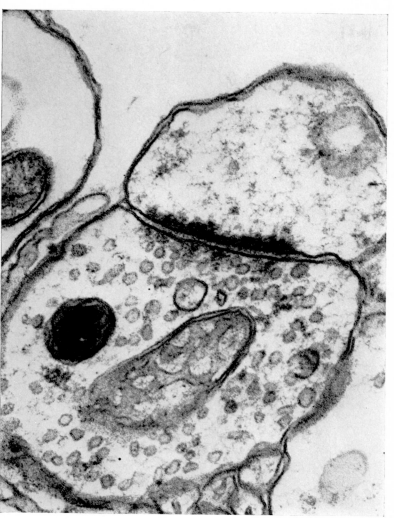

Fig. 4. A chemical synaptic connection between nerve cells of the human cerebral cortex seen by electron microscopy. The pre-synaptic terminal has many vessicles which probably contain the transmitter substance, and some other organelles. The contact with a branch of the post-synaptic cell is at the area of thickened membranes. The picture is exactly 2 μm across so the diameter of the pre-synaptic terminal is about 1 μm. (From Dr. Brian Cragg.)

The majority of intercellular connections in the brain do not function as reliable transmitters of impulses from cell to cell. Synaptic axonal terminals on post-synaptic cell membranes are usually small, of the order of 0·5 μm diameter on a cell in which the dendritic branching tree, receiving most of the synaptic connections, may extend 2000 μm. Each synaptic ending influences the conductivity of only a small patch of the post-synaptic cell membrane and the disturbance produced by transmitter action may not be sufficiently intense to generate an impulse, propagated by the whole post-synaptic cell. Firing a discharge of a nerve cell requires the concerted action of many synaptic endings and the number of these which may be found on one cell is enormous. Estimates made for the mammalian cerebral cortex reach the figure of 50 000 per cell, although not all of these may come from separate neurones. Nevertheless, the initiation of a propagated impulse in such a neurone will depend on the co-operation of a very large number of other nerve cells. To further complicate matters, the contribution of each synaptic ending to the ultimate discharge of the post-synaptic cell is not equal. In many neurones the site at which the propagated impulse appears to be generated is the region where the cell body narrows into the axon. The intensity of current flow through this region of the nerve cell has the maximum effectiveness in setting up the impulse. Activity generated close to the axonal regions will have a more marked effect on the membrane at this critical place than will activity generated at the end of a long dendritic branch, perhaps some millimeters from the axon-cell body junction. Synaptic contacts near the cell body and particularly those near the axon hillock will therefore develop an impulse more readily than will synaptic endings at the very tips of an extended dendritic tree. The synaptic input to any given cell is thus weighted in two ways; by the number of endings from any given source which can be expected to act together to influence the post-synaptic cell, and the position which those endings occupy on the cell membrane. On the remote branches of a neurone concerted action of several synaptic endings close together may on occasion generate an action potential on that branch alone. Once this has begun the electrical contribution of those synapses would become amplified by the active response of the post-synaptic membrane and the likelihood of eventual discharge of the whole cell body and axon would be correspondingly increased. It is not clear whether this mechanism is important in the integrative processes of mammalian brains. A similar mechanism occurs commonly in invertebrate neurones, some of which appear to consist of two electrically excitable regions separated by a non-excitable segment. Each half therefore acts as a physiological unit even though they are both parts of one cell.

Inhibitory synapses and their interactions

Other synaptic endings, morphologically almost indistinguishable from the kind just described, have a different effect on the post-synaptic membrane. Because they either produce a different transmitter molecule or because of differences in the chemical nature of the post-synaptic membrane, the change induced by transmitter secretion affects the permeability of some of the smaller ions more than the larger. The result is either a small increase rather than a decrease in membrane potential or no change at all. Whatever happens, the impedance of the membrane is lowered so that current flows more easily through the affected area of membrane than through the nearby resting membrane. Should an excitatory synapse have lowered the membrane potential of the same cell by setting up a depolarizing excitatory post-synaptic potential, the current flow will be channelled preferentially through the areas affected by the inhibitory synapse. Other areas of membrane will be protected from transverse current flow and the membrane potential will not be reduced as much as it would have been if the inhibitory synapse was not working. The probability that the trigger level of membrane potential necessary for production of an action potential will be reached, is therefore lowered. One cell may have very many inhibitory endings on it and presumably their effectiveness is weighted by geometry in the same way as that of the excitatory terminals.

Furthermore, there is another inhibitory mechanism of common occurrence in the brain. Some pre-synaptic terminals themselves carry synapses from other pre-synaptic cells, to form a serial synapse of two successive pre-synaptic terminals leading to one post-synaptic membrane. The effect of the first synapse in the series is to depolarize the membrane of the second terminal. But whereas the effect of this action on cell bodies is to increase the probability of firing, it has no effect on the transmission of an impulse already travelling in the second pre-synaptic cell. The lowered membrane potential of the second terminal does however lower the amount of transmitter substance released by this synapse on to the final cell. The mechanism of this is not fully understood. Nevertheless, such an action will reduce the potency of a given synaptic ending by lowering the amount of transmitter secreted, without affecting the membrane of the post-synaptic cell directly. The process is referred to as pre-synaptic inhibition to distinguish it from the post-synaptic inhibition just described. Such action may not always be inhibitory; inhibitory neurones could have sequential or serial synapses of this nature and pre-synaptic inhibition in this situation will be finally read as excitation (Eccles, 1969).

Many nerve cells have short axons that terminate in the region of the cell body. Their occurrence in the brain of all animals is as frequent, or more so, than the larger long-axon neurones that clearly transmit information from place to place. The physiology of short axon cells, called Type II neurones by Camilio Golgi, their nineteenth-century discoverer, is still largely unknown because in most instances they are too small to study by physiological methods. It is difficult to know whether such cells always or ever develop a propagated action potential, and it is possible that some of them release their transmitter more or less continuously and at a rate that is proportional to their membrane potential. It is not certain then that synaptic action in the brain is always episodic, triggered by an action potential of a few thousandths of a second's duration. Continuous release of a substance with a modulating action on adjacent cell membranes could possibly modify their response to other transmitters pulse-released on to the same membrane. There is already evidence of such interaction in peripheral synapses of the involuntary nervous system (e.g. Paton and Vizi, 1963). A more detailed account of the physiology of synapses is found in Eccles (1964).

Integration of information by synapses and neurones

Thus, nerve cells can operate as decision-making machines, the decision reached being the discharge of an action potential which depends on depolarization of the membrane, often at a critical point near the region where the axon leaves the cell body. The battle for control of membrane potential is waged according to a complex non-linear algebra in which excitatory and inhibitory synaptic actions compete by adjusting membrane permeability and current flow due to pulses of transmitter substance injected on to the cell membrane. Whether or not the cell eventually does produce an action potential depends on the number, location, relative potency, and timing of activation of excitatory and inhibitory synapses, each one the product of a similar process occurring in each pre-synaptic cell. Small wonder the mathematics of transmission in a real neurone has scarcely begun, let alone the mathematics of a network of even a few of them.

RECEPTORS

Information about the outside world and also about the state of the internal bodily organs is fed into the brain by the receptors which include distance receptor organs such as the eye, ear, and nose as well as receptors in the skin, joints, and viscera. All these receptors are connected to the brain via nerve fibres that are branches of neurones and carry pulse signals in the way that has been described. The function of the receptor organs is to transduce energy falling on the organ, be it in the form of photons, sound waves, or a mechanical indentation, and to reproduce some characteristics of the waveform of the impinging energy in the form of a graded depolarization of the tip of the receptor nerve fibre. This depolarization is called a generator potential. It acts on the adjacent membrane to produce a depolarization which, if intense enough, will activate the action potential mechanism of the sensory fibre and send an impulse up to the central nervous system. Should the generator potential remain after the first impulse departs, because of continued sensory stimulation, the adjacent membrane will produce another action potential as soon as it has recovered from the first. A train of impulses can thus be set off, the duration of which is as long as the imposed stimulus and the frequency of which is proportional to the intensity of the generator potential. All receptors function in this general way, to convert various kinds of energy to frequency-coded trains of identical impulses in their sensory neurones, the characteristics of which reflect something of the stimulus. The transduction mechanisms for dealing with light energy, sound energy, chemical sensitivities, and so on, are quite different and too intricate for full description here; but the impulses set up in the various sensory nerves are all of the same kind (Mellon, 1968).

GLIAL CELLS

Nerve cells, in the central and peripheral nervous systems, make up only about half the cellular volume of the brain. Each neurone is accompanied and partly ensheathed by another type of cell, the glial cell. These are of similar embryological origin to neurones but different electrophysiologically because they have high and stable membrane potentials and are not capable of carrying action potentials. Their function is nutritive and supporting and they are apparently not part of the signal-carrying mechanism of the brain. The metabolism of adjacent neurones and glia has been shown to be linked and their membrane potential is passively sensitive to changes in the composition of brain extracellular fluid that can be produced by intense impulse-carrying activity of the neurones. Glial cells act as intermediaries between neurones and the blood supply of the brain. They often have one process attached to the walls of the capillary blood vessels of the brain and other processes interleaving among the surrounding neurones. Neurones are unusual in that they metabolize only glucose for energy, have no auxiliary stores, and require continuous oxygen to convert glucose to CO_2. Glial cells contain an enzyme to hasten the dissociation of waste CO_2 and transport it to the blood as bicarbonate ion. They probably transport glucose, amino acids, and other metabolic building blocks to neurones for the manufacture of structural protein and enzymes necessary for transmitter synthesis and degradation (Kuffler and Nicholls, 1966).

BRAIN CODES

How, then, does this collection of about a million million cells, connected to the environment by sensory transducing organs and connected to the body muscles and glands by motor nerves, work to control something as complicated as the behaviour of man? As far as we now know, there are only two principles involved, a principle of connectivity and a principle of timing, a space code and a time code. In essence, this means that a nerve cell may carry information specified by the connection it has with other nerve cells and it may carry information by virtue of some aspect of the frequency of impulses.

Space codes

Space codes operate strongly at the input and output side of the nervous system. Each muscle in an animal can, by contraction, produce a given set of joint movements and each muscle is commanded by a group of neurones in the central nervous system that have only this function. Activity in these neurones always means, therefore, that a particular muscle will contract and that a particular set of movements will result. In lower animals this system can be shown to extend back into the nervous system. Neurones can be identified which when stimulated will cause the excitation of a set group of motoneurones which in turn will cause contraction of a set group of muscles to produce a rigidly specified movement of the whole animal. Tail flicks of crayfish for defensive swimming are controlled in this way by certain command neurones in the central nervous system of the animal. Presumably these neurones only make synaptic contact with certain rigidly specified motoneurones and transmission at these junctions is reliable. Activity in the command neurones therefore has a fixed result, co-ordinated movement of the whole tail and this occurs by virtue of the anatomical connections of the neurones. This is a system that is built entirely of space-coded neurones (Wiersma, 1947; Zucker, 1972).

In sensory systems, space codes can be recognized too. The nerve supply of mammalian skin, giving rise to the sensations of touch, pressure, heat, cold, and so on, is enormously complex. However each patch of skin can be broken down into a mosaic of points, some maximally sensitive to heat, some to light touch, and some to hair movement. Each of these modalities of sensation is signalled to the brain by a different sensory nerve fibre. The sensory neurones themselves can therefore be classified the same way as sensation, each one carrying information from a particular kind of transducing mechanism in a small patch of skin.

It takes three nerve cells to carry this information to the cerebral cortex, that is, there are two synaptic relays involved, one at the top of the spinal cord and one in the depths of the brain before fibres carrying information about cutaneous sensation emerge on to the cortical surface. It is possible to identify the cortical cells on to which these fibres now synapse by recording their electrical activity with a microscopic needle electrode.

The skin can now be explored with a fine probe to determine which kinds of stimuli affect the firing pattern of the cortical cell and the areas of skin to which it is connected. Such experiments have revealed a remarkable precision of organization of sensory pathways. Laid out on the cerebral cortex is a map of the body surface with cells that are adjacent, centrally linked to adjacent skin areas peripherally. Each cell is responsible for signalling the occurrence of some stimulus falling on a particular area of the body surface, forming a space code for the location of stimuli. Further analysis of such cells reveals that they also discriminate between kinds of stimuli applied to the skin in the same way as do the peripheral nerve fibres. Each cell responds to only one modality of skin sensation so that one which responds to light touch over a given area is not sensitive to deep pressure. One which does respond to a stimulus strong enough to distort subcutaneous structures, does not respond at all to light touch. This distinction between the kinds of stimuli to which receptors will respond is made by specializations of the receptor organ (Mountcastle, 1957).

What is important here is that this distinction is maintained from cell to cell over at least three synapses to produce populations of cortical neurones that are space-coded not only for the location of peripheral stimuli but also for the kind of stimulus. The discharge of action potentials in a given cortical neurone therefore has a double significance; it specifies both the location and the nature of a sensory stimulus. This information is coded by a rigid specificity in the formation of synapses for the peripheral nerves through the brain to the cerebral cortex.

Space coding in the visual system has been studied in even more detail (Hubel and Wiesel, 1959). Cortical neurones exist, whose discharge is governed by the position, dimensions, orientation, colour, velocity, and direction of movement of an object in the visual field. Only if all the requirements are fulfilled will the cell discharge maximally; once they are met it will respond in a perfectly stereotyped manner as many times as the stimulus is repeated. These are elaborately space-coded neurones and along the chain of nerve cells from the eye to the cerebral cortex, each successive cell makes only specified functional contacts with cells of the next stage, and each regrouping of information further restricts the range of possible sensory stimuli to which a neurone may respond. The synapses are exactly specified and they can also transmit reliably enough to always produce activity in the relevant pathway time after time.

The development of these space-coded systems is largely controlled by genetic and embryological mechanisms and the way in which they might work is discussed in Chapter 3.

Time codes

Given a specified set of connections there is another way in which information can be transmitted, which may be called the time code. One can make a distinction between two types of time code. The intensity of a stimulus is partially coded in one form. Here, a strong stimulus that evokes a large generator potential in a sense organ will initiate a high-frequency train of impulses in the sensory fibre. A smaller stimulus produces a smaller generator potential and a lower frequency of afferent nerve impulses. Frequency of impulses, or some derivative of it, therefore codes intensity of the stimulus. This form of coding has also been followed into the brain and holds true for central sensory neurones too.

The second class of time code emerges from the finding that many neurones in the central nervous system discharge impulses spontaneously, that is, in the absence of synaptic stimulation. In some cases this spontaneous activity is metabolically controlled from the cell bodies and may vary predictably with, for example, the time of day (Strumwasser, 1967). In other cases neurones are maintained at a constant level of impulse activity by random or non-patterned synaptic activity coming from other neurones or from sense organs. These, in turn, affect the impulse activity of the neurones to which they project, applying a constant excitatory or inhibitory pressure depending on the nature of the synapses they form.

The brain therefore settles into a dynamic pattern of activity which characteristically fluctuates in intensity and distribution with time. This behaviour is very characteristic of neuronal networks in many animals. The cyclic firing of neurones controlling the respiratory movements of the diaphragm and other muscles are examples of such an oscillating pattern of activity. In the cerebral cortex of man, groups of neurones fall into a recurring cycle of excitability with a much faster predominant frequency, about 10 Hz. These resting patterns become disrupted when sensory information flows into the brain.

There are experimentally defined situations where the nature of the response of part of the brain is clearly designed to fit the dynamic properties of the outflow network of neurones. Cells from the cerebellar cortex are continuously, but not regularly, active and all terminate by inhibitory synapses. The post-synaptic neurones on to which they project are therefore held in a state of constant inhibition from this source. Other synaptic inputs on the same post-synaptic neurones have predominantly excitatory connections and supply a continuous, non-patterned, excitatory input which, in spite of the concurrent inhibition, results in a 'spontaneous' discharge of 50–100 impulses per second. These cells in turn project to certain brain stem neurones which, because of synaptic convergence, receive from this latter 2500–5000 pulses of excitatory transmitter per second. This is sufficient to hold the membrane depolarized by about 10–20 mV, about one-fifth of the total membrane potential and therefore on the threshold of discharge. If now the first cell in the chain, that from the cerebellar cortex is made to fire faster, it will inhibit the next one which will in turn therefore fail to excite the third cell by simply withholding its excitatory input. The net effect on the third cell is therefore inhibition through lack of a constant facilitating input, a process known as disfacilitation. The whole effect depends on a maintained frequency of discharge of the middle neurone and this is dependent both upon continuous synaptic input and the natural characteristics of the neuronal membrane. Should either of these change, so that the average frequency of discharge of the middle cell falls, the first cell will lose control of the third cell, even though there has been no change in interneuronal connectivity (Eccles, Ito, and Szentagothai, 1967). There are many examples of these dynamic interconnections between chains of neurones and of their disruption by anaesthesia or by brain damage.

OVERALL ORGANIZATION

Because the brain is a dynamic network, its properties therefore depend on the degree of anatomical interconnection between cells, the space code, and on the ability of the neurones to maintain certain average fixed frequencies of discharge of action potentials, the time code. The properties of such a network could be modified by a change in either code.

Furthermore, every function is represented many times in the brain with different degrees of refinement. For example, basic patterns of muscle co-ordination are controlled largely by space-coded sets of neurones in the spinal cord. Modification of these patterns in accordance with information from the organs of balance comes in at the level of the brain stem at the top of the spinal cord. Precise timing of movements is mainly a function of the cerebellum and certain collections of nerve cells beneath the cerebral cortex, the basal ganglia. Movements in response to visual stimuli receive an important contribution from the midbrain. So-called voluntary movement, including the finer aspects of learned responses, come via the cerebral cortex and the most refined movements of all, differential control of discrete movements of the fingers, are organized by one special pathway from the cerebral cortex directly down to the motoneurones of the spinal cord. Any movement, learned or not, requires the orderly co-operation of all these circuits. To speak of a centre for voluntary movement is therefore not correct, even though the loss of voluntary movement is certainly the main symptom of damage to the highest level of control, i.e. certain areas of the cortex.

A similar hierarchical organization is apparent in most functions of the brain, even the most basic ones, such as the central nervous control of breathing. The whole brain in fact is a set of hierarchical systems, each level normally dependent upon the harmonious activity of other levels which either modify or control it. Experimentally isolated, a given level of control has a certain autonomy of function, for example, the spinal cord of some animals such as rats, separated from the brain, can maintain the rhythmic muscular patterns of walking. In the intact nervous system, the ability to walk still relies upon spinal cord mechanisms or sub-routines. They are not called up in a simple fashion but modified, speeded up, slowed down, suspended, and reinstated according to information available only via the sensory input into the cerebral hemispheres. This kind of organization is largely responsible for the apparent redundancy in the brain. Localized damage in one area may disrupt the function of one level of organization but the overall function may be retained with surprisingly little deficit.

The organs of balance, the vestibular system projecting via the VIIIth cranial nerve to cerebellum, spinal cord, and cortex, are normally of critical importance in posture and muscular movement. In the complete absence of the vestibular sense other interlocking systems for muscular control, using stretch information from muscles and joints or visual information from the eyes, may completely mask the deficiency in the sense of balance, until some special circumstance, such as a sudden loss of visual cues, shows it up. Therefore an equivalent change in behaviour could be produced by neurological changes at various levels of organization.

This is all that is currently known in principle about the physiology of the brain. It is a set of hierarchically organized control systems in which impulse activity and synaptic transmission follow the same laws everywhere. All sensory experience passes into the brain as a series of discrete nerve impulses in separate space coded pathways and emerge for behaviour in the form of similar impulses travelling along similarly labelled nerve fibres destined for specific muscles. Nerve cells act as mixers and selectors of appropriate response because each one gives and receives an immense number of synaptic connections, inhibitory and excitatory. Nevertheless connections are not made at random and spatial patterns of impulse activity, reflecting environmental events or muscle contraction, are detectable deep within the brain. Spontaneous activity of nerve cells is common, the frequency of which is sometimes critical for the orderly function of a nervous network. Somewhere in such a system is lying undetected, a mechanism of modification of some aspect of brain function that can permanently alter the way it works. The result of one fleeting experience is instantly recorded and remains so as a potent influence on subsequent behaviour for a lifetime of up to a hundred years.

2 *Memory*

DEFINITIONS

INTUITIVELY it is quite clear what we mean by memory and the definitions by the more introspective nineteenth-century psychologists posed no problem in the understanding. William James (1890) says 'Memory is the knowledge of a state of mind after it has already once dropped from consciousness', but he hesitates and then goes on, 'or rather it is the knowledge of an event or fact of which meantime we have not been aware, with the additional consciousness that we have thought or experienced it before'. Five pages later he rounds off his definition by saying, 'The complete exercise of memory pre-supposes two things: (1) The retention of the remembered fact. (2) Its reminiscence, recollection, reproduction or recall'.

'Do you remember or not?' It is an unequivocal question in ordinary life and can remain scientifically unequivocal in experiments on human memory. When memory can only be inferred from a change in the behaviour of man or of an animal the presence or absence of memories is no longer clear. All animals can emit behaviour that is partly instinctive, partly the result of either fatigue or heightened reactivity, partly learned and partly the result of chance. How can we decide just which aspects of behaviour depend on learning that is biologically the same as that involved in human memory? Learning is a general term for the reorganization of behaviour as a result of individual experience and the difficulty arises in deciding which kind of adaptive behaviour in animals corresponds to that which in man is associated with the formation of memories.

CLASSIFICATION OF BEHAVIOUR AND KINDS OF LEARNING

Behaviour can be assigned a cause among a fairly small number of possible causes just by classifying the behavioural repertoire of animals. It is possible to classify all acts this way, as has been done for example by Thorpe (1963), as springing from a combination of the following: instinctive or innate behaviour; habituation; associative learning; trial-and-error learning; and territorial learning including homing abilities. Many other classifications of behaviour can be made but this is a good one to begin with.

We can make a distinction first between instinctive and habitual behaviour and the other classes of associative learning. Instinct is an inherited system of co-ordinated behaviour that involves more or less rigid, inherited, releasing mechanisms. Habituation of behaviour is the relatively persistent waning of a response as the result of repeated stimulation that is not followed by any kind of reinforcement. Adaptive behaviour within these classes can occur without it being necessary to postulate that a neurological memory is necessary to the adaptation process. The occurrence of instinctive behaviour may wax and wane in intensity according to hormone levels for example. There is no need to suggest that the absence of copulation in a pregnant rat is due to the memories of the events during the preceding oestrus. She may well have memories but it is easy to show that they do not control her behaviour in this respect, whereas hormone levels do, quite clearly.

Habituation to a repeated stimulus may be easily confused with fatigue or with the adaptation of the sense organs. Thus, an animal that has become habituated to a given situation may certainly have memories of the events leading to the habituation but one cannot say that the lack of response to the situation is a matter of these memories. There are also mechanisms of attention, separable from fatigue or adaptation of sense organs, that diminish with time the effect of continuous or repeated sensory stimuli. Attention mechanisms or habituation may or may not involve learning. It is very difficult, however, to decide the relative contributions of sensory adaptation, fatigue, habituation, attention changes, and learning to the waning response to a repeated stimulus even though there are behavioural techniques for sorting out these factors (Horn and Hinde, 1970).

There remain certain behavioural situations that give rise to modifications of behaviour that can only be understood if we assume that a process very similar to human learning and memory storage has taken place within the brain of the animal.

Pavlovian conditioning

By definition there are two main classes of such associative learned behaviour, Pavlovian or classical conditioning and instrumental or operant conditioning. Pavlovian conditioning (Pavlov, 1906) involves the temporal association of two stimuli which must appear always in the same order, the conditioned (or conditional) stimulus (CS), followed by the unconditioned stimulus (UCS). The unconditioned stimulus is chosen to give a constant reliable response (UCR) from the animal without the need of training: the withdrawal of a limb from a painful stimulus, salivation in response to the taste of food, eye blink in response to a puff of air, or some such. The response to the unconditioned stimulus is known as the unconditioned response.

A particular conditioned stimulus is chosen on the grounds that it never or only very rarely elicits a response similar to the unconditioned response. If the latter is to be a flexion of the forepaw, then the sound of a buzzer or a flash of light would be suitable as a conditioned stimulus since without the conditioning procedure neither of these would be likely to be followed consistently by flexion of the forelimbs. If the response were an eye blink, then a strong flash of light could not be chosen as the conditioned stimulus because it would often evoke the blink. A weak light that did not produce reflex blinking would be quite acceptable.

Observation of conditioned reflexes is facilitated by keeping all other behaviour at bay, which is done either by previously training the animals or subjects to suppress all other reactions, or by forcibly restraining the animals so that nothing else is possible. Repeated application of the CS followed by the UCS will eventually lead to the CS eliciting a response very similar to the UCR even in the absence of the second stimulus. This is the conditioned reflex. Continued absence of the second stimulus and its consequences will eventually result in the decline of the response to the conditioned stimulus, a process known as extinction. Following a rest period the response to the conditioned stimulus can re-emerge. If extinction is not allowed to occur the response to the conditioned stimulus will remain, more or less permanently. Almost any pair of normal or artificially produced sensory stimuli may be used in Pavlovian conditioning. Involuntary responses such as slowing of the heart are as available as are voluntary responses, or artificial stimuli from direct stimulation of the brain may be used instead of stimuli applied in the normal way through the sense organs.

The time sequence of CS–UCS is critical to the establishment of conditioned reflexes. In most animals intervals of about half a second are most effective, longer intervals are less effective and, if the sequence is reversed so that the conditioned stimulus is applied after the unconditioned stimulus, learning becomes impossible or takes very much longer to become established (backward conditioning).

Operant conditioning

The other main kind of learning, instrumental or operant conditioning, differs in that a response emitted by the animal is critical to the learning. In classical conditioning it is incidental.

An animal is placed in a situation in which it will begin to explore in some way or another. If certain actions are rewarded, by food, water, or any other appropriate stimulus, the frequency of the rewarded actions increases.

The study of learning in these circumstances emerged more or less independently from the Russian school and the American school. Miller and Konorski (1928), in experiments repeated in Pavlov's laboratory, differentiated between Type II conditioning (instrumental conditioning) and Type I conditioning (Classical Pavlovian). Earlier this century, the American psychologist, Thorndike (1911) was recognizing two kinds of learning, associative shifting which corresponded to Type II and instrumental, operant, or, as he called it, Type R conditioning, which has been studied in detail by Skinner and his followers since the 1930s. Skinner designed an experiment in which a confined animal was rewarded for a particular response (Skinner, 1961). A rat in a small and otherwise featureless cage was presented with a movable bar. He pressed it and was rewarded—a piece of food dropped into the cage. A pigeon in a cage was presented with a spot. He pecked it and was rewarded with a grain of cereal. Under these conditions an animal learns very quickly to feed itself by using the rewarded action. The distinction between the two kinds of learning emphasized by Skinner is that a lever does not evoke its pressing in the sense that food evokes salivation. On the contrary, strange surroundings evoke a huge range of exploratory movements none of which are stereotyped by the environment, although they may be constrained by the limited motor repertoires of the animal. One of these acts, called an operant by Skinner, generates a reward. The effect is to increase the probability of this operant at the expense of others. Each selected operant act need not be rewarded to keep the response rate high. Reward at intervals or after so many responses serves as well or better. Continued absence of the reward, as with classical conditioning, leads to fading and ultimate loss of the operant, a process also called extinction.

The reinforcement can be an obvious one, food for a hungry animal, water for a thirsty one, or it may be a removal or reduction of an unpleasant stimulus, such as lowering of sound volume or cooling of a heated cage.

Stimuli that have no apparent rewarding function of their own can be used for reinforcement if their application is normally associated with reward. The click of a food dispenser in operation can become reinforcing even if food is not dispensed at each trial. Punishment has no place in learning of this kind. Operants are not thought to be lost as a result of punishment, although a particular response may be suppressed by punishment immediately following its execution.

It is particularly easy to produce measurable behaviour that is obviously based on learning by using operant conditioning of animals that have been deliberately deprived of food or water. A pigeon reduced by starvation to 80 per cent of its body weight and placed in an operant conditioning situation where it must peck at a target for grains of food will emit thousands of regularly spaced responses. Very precise quantitative experiments become possible, particularly on animal perception and motivation (Blough, 1958).

Reinforcement, in the simple sense of some stimulus that indicates the satisfaction of an immediate bodily need, is thought to be a necessary part of this learning process. Learning therefore has been considered as the reassortment of an animal's possible behavioural responses so as to minimize certain internal signals that indicate a physiological imbalance, such as the lack of food, water, heat, or unsatisfied sexual requirements. Such signals are known as drives and drive-reduction theories of learning have been erected in which learning affects behaviour in proportion to the results fed back to a hypothetical comparator that detects the error between an internal standard of the correct amount of drive and the change produced by any behavioural act.

The concept of arousal has been used the same way in learning theories, the idea being that there is some optimal level of arousal generated by the sum total of immediate sensory stimuli, and that the animal constantly adjusts its behaviour away from extremes. Such theories are very powerful for explaining the facts of learning experiments mostly because the explanatory concepts of drive, arousal, or curiosity are defined by the experiments they are invoked to explain. A theory involving an optimum of some internal property that cannot be measured independently may encompass anything (Berlyne, 1960).

Latent learning

A separate category may be made to include learning that does not easily fit into either of these first two groups but which is perhaps of the greatest importance in the behaviour of most animals. This is latent learning or place learning and includes homing abilities and other forms of compass navigation. Many animals behave as if they learned the geographical features of their environment by simply experiencing it without any obvious reward. The layout of escape routes to and from a lair, the recognition of a nest site of many creatures from birds to bees and solitary wasps depend on highly developed learning abilities.

The process can be brought into the laboratory where it can be shown that rats having unrewarded familiarity with a maze subsequently learn to solve the maze for reward faster than animals without prior exposure (Hilgard and Bower, 1966). Similar conclusions come from experiments using an inappropriate reward in maze learning. If rats that are hungry but not thirsty, encounter water at one place in a maze when running for food reward they will find it again much faster when reintroduced to the same maze after being fed but deprived of water.

Whether or not some latent reinforcement process is at work in this kind of learning is a matter of argument. It seems more economical to assume that mere contiguity of novel sequences of stimuli or acts is sufficient to set up a learning process, a theory which is psychologically respectable (Guthrie, 1959). It comes to almost the same thing to postulate that novel stimulus sequences themselves set up a reinforcement process that serves to link them together in time.

CONTRIBUTION OF VARIOUS KINDS OF LEARNING
TO BEHAVIOUR

The broadest and simplest classification of learned behaviour includes these three types. Pavlovian conditioning in which repeated pairing of two sensory stimuli in an otherwise passive animal leads to a change in response to the first of the pair, operant conditioning in which the frequency of occurrence of certain motor patterns in behaviour is regulated by their consequences and latent learning in which a series of sensori–motor sequences, in the absence of any obvious reward, builds up new and flexible behaviour patterns to fit an animal on to its geographical environment. This is obviously of as great a biological significance as the other two types.

None of these kinds of learning has any reality other than descriptive and had the history of experimental psychology been different quite different categories might have emerged. It is easy to find scholars who will make many additional subclassifications and others who will have no truck with the distinctions made here and refuse to see a workable separation between Pavlovian and operant conditioning. How, for example, should one classify observational learning? Many animals, and Man to a high degree, may acquire behaviour by watching others perform. Is this a form of latent learning, a form of internalized operant conditioning where both the operant and reinforcement are associated in a symbolic form in the brain, or is it a separate category?

Even the simplest learned behavioural acts must be made up of varying contributions from the various kinds of learning. The purest laboratory experiment becomes so not because the learning situation is pure but because the recording process only reveals one aspect of learning. Most experiments are mixed. An animal is placed in a cage with two identical compartments; some inocuous signal (a buzzer or light) is turned on and some seconds later some kind of punishment is administered, electrification of the floor being the most frequent. The animal may escape the shock by leaving the compartment for the opposite one where, after a rest period, the same sequence is repeated and it can be escaped by returning to the original compartment.

Placed in such a situation an animal will explore, or not, depending on the state of motivation, the time of day, hormonal levels, and other factors. Latent learning will occur. On presentation of the warning stimulus followed by the shock a Pavlovian conditioned reflex will be set up and can be measured by the occurrence of emotional defecation in response to the first stimulus, effects on heart and respiration rate, or by a somatic conditioned emotional response in which the animal simply becomes immobile. If this is overcome and the animal can begin to emit further behavioural responses or operants, one of these, leaving one compartment for the other, terminates the shock. The operant is therefore strengthened. With repeated presentations most animals pass through a stage where their operant learning enables them to escape each shock as it begins and enter a stage where they can avoid the shock completely by leaving the compartment on presentation of the conditioned stimulus. This is now called avoidance conditioning.

Each learning situation, coupled with the chosen recording technique throws one aspect of learning into prominence.

From classical conditioning experiments the importance of timing between two contiguous sensory stimuli needed for learning becomes clear. Operant experiments demonstrate the importance of a reward relevant to the motivation and state in persuading animals to base their behaviour on recent learning rather than other behavioural patterns. From latent learning experiments the complexity speed and enormous capacity of learning mechanisms in the simplest of animals are only too apparent.

Experiments on whole animals reveal learning only through a change in behaviour. The commonly used learning situations, or paradigms, are designed mainly to give clear behavioural indices of learning. Strong reinforcement used in some operant experiments becomes a way of communicating to the animal that of all its immense behavioural repertoire only certain recently learned acts are useful in the present circumstances. Such a flexibility of behavioural resources whereby the springs of behaviour can be adjusted according to current pay-off must have some physiological mechanism.

However, the notion of a so-called reinforcing signal, generated in the brain by the satisfactory outcome of a behavioural act and then modifying the central nervous circuits that led up to the desired event, is by no means the only way of thinking about the physiological mechanism. Other equally attractive formulations are possible (Bolles, 1972). For example, the motivating force in the brain, signifying, say, the need for food may throw the whole of the machinery of behaviour into a state of expectancy for food. This would apply to the earliest stages if the perceptual process and to exploratory tendencies necessary for finding food as well as to the consumatory responses of eating and its sensory and metabolic consequences. With the brain in such a state only certain behavioural patterns become relevant and those most likely to occur are the ones that take the animal right through from the first sensory hints of food to the final metabolic relief. These responses therefore occur in preference to other responses that are blocked in their run to completion, as defined by the hungry brain, so that mere repetition becomes the requirement for learning. If psychological theory can encompass the mechanism of learning by this idea of expectancy and incentive motivation as well as by the idea of a reinforcing signal which validates the immediately preceding behaviour, we have no more right to look for a reinforcing neuronal system than an expectancy neuronal system (Kety, 1972).

This problem occurs over and over again in theoretical writing about the logical requirements of learning neuronal circuits, as well as in the kind of thinking used to set up physiological experiments on possible mechanisms of learning. It is not reasonable to abstract the verbal or logical representation of each component of a particular behavioural situation that can be used to demonstrate learning and then demand a physiological explanation for all these abstractations at the same biological level. Yet many physiologically inclined workers have simply taken each of the parameters of a conventionally accepted learning paradigm such as classical conditioning and assumed that there is a cellular explanation for each of them.

In contrast, those intimately concerned with learning theories, the psychologists, knowing the complexity of the situations that they are trying to describe, tend to hold their theories more to create arguments that may deepen understanding than to defend an entrenched position. One or other theory still gains ascendancy by historical accident or force of personality, by a process that is more literary or philosophical than scientific. Unlike the physical sciences, as psychology progresses more and more theories come to coexist, the newest not entirely replacing the older ones because each represents a valid viewpoint that is not destroyed by more recent insights. The fault is on the side of the supposedly analytical physiologist or biochemist, even anatomist, who is prepared to take the behavioural data as it comes and on occasions as a rather easy option, something that can be picked up on the side (Hebb, 1958; Krech, 1972).

THE DETECTION OF MEMORY

Once a behavioural change has been induced by environmental manipulation it cannot be attributed to permanent memory formation unless it lasts a long time and may be re-evoked under the appropriate circumstances. This means that the behavioural method for detecting the memory must disclose this particular cause for behaviour rather than any other.

Traditionally there are three methods for doing this, the methods of recall, recognition, and relearning. These categories came from experiments on human verbal learning but in general are applicable to animal experiments as well.

Recall involves the complete replay of acquired behaviour from minimal cues in the test situation. With man it is simply a matter of saying, 'Please write down the list of words you learned yesterday.' With animals we understand less about the subtleties of their communication and it is not so easy to give sufficient cues as to the required behaviour without giving the whole thing away. The method therefore shades off into that of recognition, in which the previous environmental stimulus situation is presented in full and the subsequent behaviour recorded. Clearer indices of learning are available if there is some kind of choice involved on the animals' part. Two visual stimuli varying in some predetermined dimension may be placed at different parts of the test cage, only one of which is associated with the previous reward or punishment. Relearning involves the updating of learned behaviour in the test situation. It may be a continuation of the previous learning with reinforcement given as before, it may measure the degree of persistence of behaviour when the reinforcement is withheld, the method of extinction, or reinforcement contingencies may be reversed so that learning of an opposing response must be superimposed upon the previous learning, which is the method of reversal learning.

Then there is the matter of the kind of response required to reveal learning and the criteria adopted by the experimenter as to its success or failure. In the first place the response may be active or passive. The animal may seek out the appropriate stimulus in an exploratory manner or it may reveal learning by withholding an exploratory tendency. In the recognition method stimuli may be presented together, in which case a choice between them will be required, or they may be presented sequentially in which case the choice becomes whether to respond or not to respond. The experimenter may measure learning in the latter situation by the time elapsed between presentation of the stimulus and the emergence of the response, on the assumption that longer latencies signify weaker learning.

Since the behaviour of the experimental animal is controlled by many factors, other than the particular known learning in the past, the nature of the method of testing will be of importance in whether or not the memory shows up. For example the training situation, which is usually a strong and unique experience in the life of the animal, may induce general emotional effects on subsequent behaviour. This may be a heightened reactivity or a tendency to passivity. In the memory test a heightened reactivity in a passive response situation will be antagonistic to the learned response, a tendency to passivity or freezing will be additive. These general effects may completely overlay the specific learned response and be measured as memory retention, or the lack of it, unless some careful behavioural controls are carried out. Sensitization or pseudo-conditioning is interesting as a mechanism of behaviour in its own right. In experiments on the cellular nature of the specific memory store such effects must be constantly watched for and eliminated by the correct experimental design.

Retrieval of memory is thus as critical a technical problem as is the method of its induction. Once again there is no firm ground. If acquired behaviour does not show up on retest one must try and discover the mechanism. The first question is whether the registration has failed or whether retrieval is impaired.

The perceptive study of behaviour is a necessary part of memory research because, after all, the behavioural change in the phenomenon under investigation. We cannot expect the methods of experimental psychology or animal behaviour to define the conditions for memory formation or to be completely reliable as assays of formed memory. Thoughts as to the possible physiological mechanism are more likely to come from the analytical study of neurophysiology and brain development, than from the increasingly refined analysis of behaviour.

POSSIBLE CORRELATES OF LEARNING IN NERVE CELLS

In looking for a mechanism of learning at the level of cell biology one must look first for the simplest common feature of learning in all situations. What can be extracted from these situations that is quite indispensable for learning, and how much of this can be rephrased in terms of the cell biology of neurones, as it is now understood? This is the problem that at present would be most useful to solve. These are terribly tight limits and it seems on first sight that nothing can be done. We cannot look directly, for example, for the physiological mechanism of the conditioned reflex, because at the moment it may not exist among the neurones in a comprehensible form. Also, from the neurophysiological summary of Chapter 1, which though brief is not unduly harsh, nothing that is easily matched with psychologically useful ideas springs to mind.

At the very least an event must be experienced to be learned. Information must come into the nervous system, which means that a characteristic pattern of nerve impulses must be set up. That pattern must leave a trace which is capable of becoming the substrate for memory. All sensory stimulation, natural, via any one or a combination of the senses, or unnatural, via electrical stimulation of the brain, has this potentiality.

The trace must be different in kind or intensity from the initial pattern. Neither perceptions nor motor acts that become memories persist in themselves, but are quickly overlaid by subsequent sensory messages or motor behaviour and the recurrence of a past pattern easily recognized. Whether or not the initial trace becomes a memory depends upon other events in the nervous system. Some things are learned apparently only because they are new, as in latent learning or place learning, some things because of repetition as in operant conditioning and some perhaps because of subsequent reactions of the nervous system as in the formation of classical conditioned reflexes. One might expect therefore that the initial trace should last at least long enough to span the interval between a conditioned stimulus and the unconditioned stimulus that follows, or between an operant and its sensory consequences. This is not much of a constraint because these intervals are best kept as short as possible in behavioural experiments, about 0.5 s.

The brevity of the optimal interval between stimulus and reinforcement or unconditioned stimulus is such as to suggest that the two patterns of neuronal activity may very well interact while both in the nerve impulse code and that memory is stored by a trace developing in only those nerve cells whose activity requires the correctly ordered temporal association of two stimuli.

However, since much learning occurs with no apparent motivation it is not necessary on behavioural grounds to include a mechanism of reinforcement or drive reduction in either psychological learning theories or in the most limited cellular hypothesis of memory.

The problem therefore is reduced to finding a neuronal consequence of sensory stimulation that can and sometimes does become converted into a permanent change. Since the most rapid and biologically useful learning occurs in relation to perception of the whole environment, one would expect it to occur best at a level in the nervous system where the simultaneous input from a variety of sense organs can come together and exert a mutual influence upon the selection of appropriate motor responding. This occurs at the highest organizational level in the nervous system where integration of visual, olfactory, somesthetic and other senses is possible.

So far it is only here that the large amount of psychological work on human learning, specially of verbal material, can be brought into a physiological context. It is now clear that information entering the human brain tumbles through a series of filtering and encoding processes before the residue comes to rest in a form that may be converted into permanent memory. The preliminary processes take time, a few seconds or perhaps minutes under special circumstances, during which the information remains available for the direction of behaviour even though its coding is altering. This stage of information storage is known as psychological short-term memory and contains at least two recognizable stages, and perhaps could be described as containing more if the complexity of material and that of the behavioural situation was increased (Broadbent, 1970; but see Craik and Lockhart, 1972). Once information is in the psychological long-term phase there is physiological evidence that the physical mechanism of storage may slowly change over longer times, minutes to hours, and this is dealt with in Chapter 4.

The importance of the discovery of the short-term psychological memory process was to emphasize that the raw material for permanent memory exists in the human brain in a different code than that of the primary perceptions. Therefore it must be stored at a different level of organization in the brain corresponding perhaps to the code for planning motor responses on the basis of the whole of the sensory input rather than that for sensation. It would be very hazardous to suggest that this level of organization corresponded to any anatomical subdivision of the brain, such as the cerebral cortex, because we know that the cortex does not function without its hierarchical connections with the rest of the nervous system. Therefore there is no reason, from this kind of evidence, to expect the learning abilities of nerve cells to be confined to any particular neuronal structure. There is evidence to remove the learning neurones out of the direct pathways from the sense organs and to suggest that human learning consists of more than the direct replay of sensation.

From this point of view the central physiological problem of memory becomes much less daunting. Nerve cells are not all that complicated, or physiologically diverse, and the common consequences of their electrical activity are not very difficult to measure or to study, electrically, or biochemically. Knowing the principles of the development, anatomy, physiology, and biochemistry of the brain, which of these known changes as they occur, more or less, in all neurons would be the best candidate as a mechanism of permanent change?

THE USE OF LEARNING EXPERIMENTS

In studying learning at this level there is no need to go into the question of the nature of the coded information, the relation of these experimental approaches on animals to human verbal or motor learning, or to the purely psychological issues of stimulus—response theories of learning versus cognitive theories. Perhaps the only lesson to keep in mind is the extraordinary rapidity and capacity of human learning, particularly of verbal learning. Pavlov coped with this problem by assigning language to a second signalling system in the brain of man, immeasurably more powerful and precise than the primary system of the conditioned reflex. This is still a useful distinction because it suggests that the use of language depends on the elaboration of a new coding and calculating system in the evolving cerebral cortex. We are not driven to postulate anything new about the properties of the individual human neurones nor of their biophysical or biochemical mechanisms. Different coding systems in nerve nets of varying connectivity may conceal or enhance the effect that a small change in neuronal properties may have on influencing the outcome of impulse activity in the net. Whatever the system, manipulation of the mechanism whereby nerve cell properties are changed and therefore memories are retained, will be recognizable in the behaviour of the ensemble.

At the moment we lack the technical ability to reveal the constantly changing patterns of brain activity that underlie the behaviour of even the simplest animals, let alone man. Even if we could demonstrate such a pattern we probably lack the descriptive or mathematical methods for its understanding. Such limitations force us back to the most basic physiology of the nerve cell as the only possible level at which to attack the biological problem of neurological memory. Even when we discover the crucial cellular mechanism we may still be at a loss to explain how this might affect the function of nerve cell networks.

It is possible therefore to study memory while not knowing what is learned nor why it is learned. Obviously the various conditioning procedures like those described in this chapter by no means define the conditions in which learning can occur. They do define certain conditions in which the behaviour of an animal can be made to depend upon learning and this is their empirical usefulness. The experimenter is therefore dependent on the various tried psychological paradigms in designing experiments on the neurological basis of learning and memory. Whether one experiments with a whole animal or an isolated piece of the nervous system they provide tools for the detection of learning and memory. Furthermore, the degree to which any newly found biological mechanisms can account for the known features of the various conditioning procedures provides an initial screen through which any theory must pass.

3 Neuroembryology

THE behaviour of animals is adapted for a very large number of different habitats, kinds of food, and ways of life. The most universal behaviours, however, those associated with breathing, the mechanisms of eating and drinking, conservation of body heat, are so similar from animal to animal that within a species it is reasonable to believe that such functions are inherited as complete units. Instinct was the term used to describe these and other common and vital aspects of behaviour and the word came unfortunately to have explanatory and satisfying overtones that for a long time impeded further analytical thought about the brain mechanisms involved. The concept, towards the end of the last century, was extended in a most unproductive way to provide an instinct for self-preservation, maternity, aggression, and so on, until the whole of observable animal behaviour became simply a series of interlocking instincts, selected of course by environmental pressures and following the principles of evolution, but instincts nevertheless (Beach, 1955).

Obviously for man and for any domestic or laboratory animal, the behaviour of which is known in detail, such an explanation or description is not adequate because individuals vary widely in their responses to standard situations. Furthermore they are adaptable and will modify behaviour, which originally might have been classed as instinctive according to its success. How much behaviour therefore is instinctive, and how much is acquired by practice and experience, how much heredity, how much environment, how much nature, how much nurture? These are useful questions about the mechanism of behaviour in that they force the question back to the physiology of the nervous system. To what extent are the actions of animals fixed by the nature of the inherited and embryologically determined forces acting in brain development and to what extent may these actions be modified by experience? Since animals do vary widely in their behavioural capabilities, is this because their brains are developmentally programmed during embryonic growth with the precise nervous networks that will be necessary for dealing with their future life, or does the development of the brain leave them largely an empty and uncommitted computer which will allow them to develop behaviour patterns adequate for survival of the species.

There is no one answer to this, because each question dealing with a particular aspect of behaviour in a certain animal needs a separate and detailed reply. There do emerge, however, certain principles that are of great relevance to the problem of memory. The matter to be considered in this chapter is that aspect of neuroembryology that might bear upon the development and modifiability of instinctive behaviour. It is as well to realize at the outset that there are no satisfactory neurological explanations for behavioural acts in the higher vertebrates, even though good progress has been made recently with simple invertebrates. This does not matter because, as in the considerations of the moment-to-moment physiology of nerve cells, we are only looking for principles that will help to make sense of matters of immense complexity that are still mainly beyond the capacities of scientific description.

THE SHAPE OF THE BRAIN

The early embryologists dealt with the development of the nervous system just as with the other organs of the vertebrate body, and described its changing shape at various stages from fertilization to adult (Harrison, 1935). The development of the vertebrate brain begins very early on, as a strip of ectodermal cells from the outer covering of the embryo and sharing the same origin as the skin of the adult. Along the dorsal surface of the embryo a plate of cells becomes recognizable as the precursor of the brain and is known as the neural plate, or neurectoderm. These cells proliferate more rapidly than the surrounding ectodermal cells and come to form a depression and then a groove, wider and deeper anteriorly but extending the length of the embryo to the tail. The edges of the groove grow together and seal progressively from front to back. Eventually the tube formed this way becomes separate from the overlying ectoderm. The central nervous system develops by expanding and folding of the original tube. The central cavity is retained through life and is present as a fine canal through the spinal cord, which retains its tubular structure. The brain develops certain large swellings. The cerebellum in the midline just above the spinal cord grows from the roof of the neural tube and is a solid structure that overlies the central canal, which continues up through the brain stem. The anterior blind end of the neural tube grows two symmetrical lateral outpouchings which expand enormously in the higher vertebrates and come to form the cerebral hemispheres, which although densely folded and convoluted, are still hollow and retain their central ventricles connecting to the central canal of the nervous system. The interconnecting canals and ventricles contain the clear cerebrospinal fluid which also bathes the outer surface of the brain and the two fluid-filled compartments connect by a small hole in the dorsal surface of the brain stem just behind the cerebellum.

The core of the vertebrate brain is common to most animals. From the spinal cord up to the areas of the mid-brain controlling the movements of the eyes, and including centres for projection of the optic and auditory nerves and the areas concerned with respiration, cardiovascular regulation, and other very basic functions, very little difference is known to exist in the organization of neurones in these areas from sharks to man. The differences in brain structure that are most pronounced are in the progressive development of the forebrain and particularly the cerebral hemispheres in higher vertebrates and man (Kappers, Huber, and Crosby, 1960). The gross shape of the brain is determined by cell division, migration, and cell death just as in other organs of the body. The relatively huge expanse of the mammalian cerebral cortex for example, is formed through prolonged and rapid multiplication of cells in certain parts of the lateral walls of the anterior end of the neural tube. These morphogenetic divisions are controlled by embryological mechanisms that must be quite similar to those forming other organs of a particular shape and size. They do not depend upon function of the organ because all the development takes place before function commences.

BRAIN FINE STRUCTURE

The development of all areas of the brain differs from that of the liver and kidney, even in those core structures common to most animals, in that its fine structure becomes quite different from region to region. There is no multicellular functional unit of the brain that is repeated throughout, as the lobule of the liver or the kidney nephron is repeated to make up a functioning whole of the required capacity. Neurones from different regions of the brain differ vastly in all respects except their unicellular nature, excitable membranes, and capacity to secrete or respond to specific chemical transmitter substances. In other structural and biochemical respects nerve cells come in a fantastic variety.

Certain fixing and staining techniques for histological examination of the nervous system, derived from the method perfected by Golgi at the end of the nineteenth century, can pick out and stain an entire neurone in isolation from its neighbours. Such prepatations clearly showed, in the hands of the histologist Cajal (1955), that the nerve cells from different parts of the brain show quite characteristic specializations in shape as well as in the connections they appeared to make by synapses with other neurones. Much of Cajal's enormously detailed and comprehensive analysis of the neuronal architecture of the mammalian brain was carried out on foetal or new-born animals (1960) so there is once again no question of experience being of prime importance in the specific determination of nerve cell shape. Additional embryological forces of a precision and complexity that far exceed those required for the formation of other organs must control the membrane outgrowths of individual nerve cells.

The idea of the uniqueness and specificity of different classes of neurones from different regions of the brain is one of the strongest general messages from Cajal's detailed investigations and that this must stem from very precise developmental control of the cellular structure of the nervous system was also recognized by him. Even within one area, the cerebral cortex for example, there are many recognizably different cell types arranged in identifiable layers with the cell bodies containing the nuclei embedded in a mesh work of fine processes coming from thousands of similar or different cell types. The detailed connections between these various types are also precisely specified so that by patient study of anatomical preparations the neuronal circuit diagrams for small areas of the brain may be pieced together. Cajal did make appreciable progress in this, although at tne time his findings did not help very much in understanding the functional circuitry because he could not tell which connections were excitatory and which were inhibitory. All his proposed circuits were of excitatory connections.

In addition to the geometrical specificity that is complex enough, more recent work showed that neurones that look much alike differ in the kind of transmitter they secrete and perhaps in other biochemical and metabolic characteristics. The nature of transmitter is also a developmentally determined and invariant feature of neurones (Dale, 1934), so an unknown number of biochemical specificities must be added to the already large number of morphological specificities required for the growth and development of the brain.

NEURONAL INDIVIDUALITY

It came as something of a shock in the late 1930s when it was demonstrated that even neurones that are morphologically identical and presumably secrete the same transmitter, differ among themselves with regard to their place in a developmental sequence. Such differences are not yet apparent in study of the brain in its mature form by anatomical, physiological, or biochemical methods. The realization that inherent differences must exist between nerve cells that are identical in all other respects came from study of the mechanism of repair of the nervous system of lower vertebrates, after surgical damage to the brain or nerves.

It had been known since the work of Waller in England in 1850 that if a nerve fibre was cut through, the part of the fibre furthest from the brain died, while the nerve stump remained healthy. Eventually a nerve became reconstituted; the paralysis and anaesthesia that had followed cutting the nerves was not permanent. Controversy raged around the mechanism of nerve repair, some maintaining that in development and in repair nerve fibres are formed by the fusion of a chain of more primitive cells, and others believing that the whole of the nerve is formed by an outgrowth of an immensely long process from the trophic centre, or nerve cell body. The matter was not easily settled. Striated muscle fibres quite definitely are formed by fusion of cells in a long chain. Nerve fibres often looked similar because early histological methods stained the sheath cells or Schwann cells that accompany all nerve fibres and in the periphery they are arranged in a chain-like manner along the fibre.

Nerve fibres do emerge from cell bodies as a continuous filament and this was shown in two ways. The most direct was an experiment performed by Ross Harrison (1910), for which he invented the technique of tissue-culture. Fragments of brain tissue, kept in a nutrient medium and observed with a microscope, could be seen to put out processes that were obviously the same as nerve fibres and which grew continually at the tip. The other evidence came again from histological observations on regenerating nerves by Cajal (1959). His silver stains for impregnating nerve fibres and the better microscopy, available by the early years of this century, gave him no doubt that cut nerves were reconstituted by growth from the central stump. He was able to show that the peripheral stump, separated from the neuronal cell bodies, became composed entirely of the satellite cells and that these even grew back a little to extend the stump towards the other cut end. Nerve trunks composed of only satellite cells did not relieve paralysis or anaesthesia and only when the fine process of the neurones grew out from the central stump, found their way into the peripheral stump, and grew down to make contact with the peripheral tissues again did function recover.

Cajal gave some attention to how the growing sprouts could find their way to the peripheral stump, even over distances of several millimetres. He noticed that nerves grew very well in among the satellite cells and also in embryonic tissues particularly of mesodermal origin. From such observations he

derived a theory of neurotropism, that the peripheral stump
may secrete chemical substances, enzymes, or the like, that
would facilitate growth, or perhaps even attract sprouts from
the central stump. He also noted that nerve fibres when they
arrived at the peripheral tissues often innervated structures
there in the same way as before. He therefore postulated a
series of more precise trophic influences that could attract the
exact nerve to the end-organ. His methods were strong in the
detail they revealed about the whole nervous structure of the
body. They were weak in that they were static and the march
of events in regeneration could only be reconstructed by a
series of stills. Neurotrophisms, general and specific, were
raised as a working hypothesis but even though the end results
revealed a good deal of specificity, he had no evidence as to the
mechanism by which this was achieved.

Individuality of muscles and their nerves

During this period of work on the origin of peripheral nerve
fibres it had been discovered that the tailed amphibians, salamanders, were unusual among the vertebrates in that a whole
limb could be grafted on to the trunk of a host animal, become
vascularized and be reinnervated by nerves which connected
to the spinal cord of the host. Paul Weiss in Vienna took up
this finding twenty years later (Weiss, 1926) and reported that
such grafted limbs not only became reinnervated by the host
but began to move in time with the adjacent host limb. The
unison of movement of the newly grafted limb and the
original limb of the host just beside it, impressed Weiss deeply
and he realized that this must indicate some very precise link-
up between the musculature of the new limb and the central
nervous system controlling the extremities. He realized that
the co-ordination could not be learned because homologous
movement of the new limb continued even if it was grafted
in an orientation that made it work against the direction of
action of the other four limbs. The reconnection of nerve and
muscle had therefore to be due to inherent growth forces in
the host and foreign tissues.

When the nerve supply of such limbs was dissected it did not
correspond precisely to that of the normal limb, which made
Weiss think that the innervation was, in fact, random. There

was nothing for it but to postulate that the foreign muscles had sent some message back through the nerves to readjust the firing pattern of nerve cell bodies, so that the pattern became appropriate for this muscle. The appropriateness depended upon the developmental origin of the muscle and its place in the limb, not upon the functional role it played in its new position on a foreign animal. This process he named myotopic modulation of motoneurones and some ingenious theories were developed by him to try and understand how it might happen (Weiss, 1931).

The important contribution by Weiss, which began a whole new line of thinking about the nervous system, was not in the details of the theory, which have since been proven wrong (Cass, Sutton, and Mark, 1973), but in the realization that some kind of precise signal, of developmental and not functional nature, must have been exchanged between the set of muscles on the one hand and the set of motoneurones and their dependent nerve fibres on the other. Each muscle cell must be marked as different from cells in other limb muscles in a way that nerve cells can recognize and vice versa.

Corresponding sets of neurones in the brain

Evidence that this principle applies to connections between neurones in the central nervous system came from a set of experiments by Sperry, who was once a student of Weiss. The optic nerve of amphibans will also regenerate when cut, just as well the peripheral nerves of the body (Stone, 1944). In these eyes, as in all vertebrates, the retina is a multi-layered structure with the light-sensitive cells forming synapses with several interneurones before the final cell which sends a very long axon through the optic nerve to the visual centres of the brain. The structure of the retina is similar all over and there is no qualitative difference between the final ganglion cells from different parts of the retina. There is, however, a difference in central connections of ganglion cells. In amphibia and fishes they terminate mainly in the mid-brain on the optic lobe (or optic tectum) and the terminations are spatially organized so that the centre of the retina projects to the centre of the tectum and peripheral points are arranged around about, in just the same order as in the retina.

The tectum is also an important region for the control of movement of the eyes and of the whole animal. There is a large bundle of fibres which leave the tectum on each side and pass down to the brain stem where they synapse with other neurones that eventually control the firing of motoneurones for the muscles which move the eyes and other body musculature. This can also be shown by electrical stimulation experiments. If a weak current is passed through a point on the surface of the optic lobe there will be movements of the eyes and body. Each region of the surface when stimulated will make the eyes and body move in a different direction (Akert, 1949).

Thus, there is a topographically precise projection from the retina on to the tectum so that the spatial arrangement of the retina is reproduced over the tectal surface and there is also a spatially discrete motor system in the mid-brain where a localized region of the tectum can be excited to cause movement of the eyes and body in a specified direction. The significance of these two superimposed maps, one sensory and one motor is the following. When an object is above the direction of gaze of the eye its image will fall on the lower half of the retina. This will send impulses up the optic nerve to produce an area of excitation in the appropriate neurones of the mid-brain. The motor outflow neurones will discharge and raise first the eyes and then the head and body so that the image of the object is moved on to the centre of the retina. It is so for other regions of the retina too. Stimulation of the tectal surface brings about movements of the eyes and head that move the retina so that the corresponding image sweeps across to the central fixation point in the eyes. The spatial organization of the projection from retinal ganglion cells to the mid-brain is therefore critical for visuomotor reactions involved in localizing objects in the visual world relative to the animal.

When the optic nerve is cut the central ends of the fibres are separated from their cell bodies in the retina and they degenerate and are replaced by satellite cells, just as in peripheral nerve. The stumps begin to grow again out from the eye and back along the course of the optic nerve to the brain. Animals become blind while this is happening, but after an interval of weeks or months, vision begins to return. When it does, the directional aspects of visual behaviour, responses to a discrete object in a particular place in the visual field, are correct from the first moment they are apparent. Full vision returns eventually, with visual acuity and colour discrimination approaching or equalling that attained by the original development (Sperry and Arora, 1963; Weiler, 1966).

Sperry's crucial experiments in the early 1940s began by

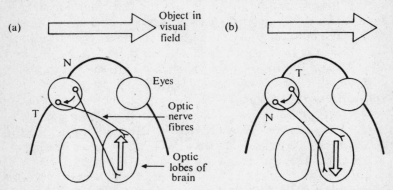

Fig. 5. The normal projection of the visual field on to the optic lobe of lower vertebrates and the effect of inverting the eye. Objects on the right of the visual field, as shown by the arrowhead, which normally cause excitation of the front of the tectum (*a*) now cause excitation at the back (*b*). Optic nerve cells from the anterior and posterior edges of the eye are labelled N (nasal) and T (temporal) in accordance with the convention usually adopted in describing the retina and visual fields.

repeating these observations with the eye mechanically inverted in the orbit so the dorsal pole was now ventral and the anterior pole posterior, which can be simply achieved in an animal with a reasonably long optic nerve by cutting eye muscles, rotating the eye 180° in the orbit and sticking it there. As soon as this is done all the visuomotor reactions of the animals (salamanders were used in the first case) reverse and remain that way for ever. Objects below the eye now form an image on the top part of the retina but the corresponding messages are transmitted to the area of the mid-brain optic lobe that used to receive messages signifying objects above the eye. The motor response, therefore, is towards the expected location above the animal, so it will strike upwards for food presented below. All visuomotor behaviour and all reflexes of visual origin are similarly reversed (Fig. 5) (Sperry, 1943a).

In spite of the ridiculously maladaptive behaviour, animals such as fish, frog, and salamanders can be kept alive by forced feeding for years in this condition and they never learn or compensate in any specific way for their disability. Sperry then cut the optic nerve in a series of salamanders with inverted eyes and waited for the regeneration of optic nerve fibres and the return of vision. In what, in retrospect at least, was one of the pivotal moments in brain research he one day offered one of his salamanders its morning piece of food, held in a pair of forceps above its head and saw the animal lunge forward and thump its chin on the ground. From then on the reversed reflexes and prey-catching behaviour emerged into the full picture shown by an animal with inverted eyes and a neurologically intact optic system (Sperry, 1943b).

Embryological determination of neural connections

The inference from this and many comparable experiments was that the terminals of optic nerve fibres had made connections in the brain according to the spatial origin of the fibres from the retina and not according to what was useful under the new circumstances. Therefore there had to have been some developmental match, between the nerve cells of the retina that gave rise to the fibres of the optic nerve, and the corresponding set of nerve cells in the optic lobe that receive synaptic connections from the retina. The developmental characters had been maintained into adult life and survived denervation and regeneration of nerve axons to direct synapse formation once again in the course of nerve repair.

If such mechanisms were so powerful in specifying connections in the face of urgent behavioural needs for a quite different pattern, several questions immediately arose: how general was this mechanism in neurogenesis; what was the nature of the developmental match between corresponding sets of otherwise identical nerve cells and how did such information become incorporated into them.

The first was satisfied by doing similar experiments on central nervous neurones mediating visuomotor co-ordination and finding that complete section of the brain stem below the tectum, which interrupts the tectal output pathway, can repair itself just as well (Sperry, 1948), as can the spinal cord of fish (Bernstein and Geldred, 1970). Similar experiments on the vestibular (Sperry, 1945, Hibbard, 1964, 1965) and olfactory pathways (Westerman, 1965) have now been done, all with the same kind of result. Nerve cross-union and skin-grafting experiments in tadpoles showed that cutaneous sensory nerve fibres also seen to make central connections appropriate for the embryological origin of the skin rather than its location on the body (Miner, 1956), in ways that are exactly reminiscent of optic nerve connections (Jacobson and Baker, 1969; Baker and Jacobson, 1970).

The only remaining discontinuity appeared to be in the formation of connections to muscles from the motoneurones of the brain stem and spinal cord. In spite of the obvious importance of precise connections between nerve cells and the corresponding muscles the evidence, until recently, was that such connections, in contrast to all others, could form at random. Co-ordination would be re-established by a reverse influence of muscle upon the motoneurone that was postulated to force it to exchange the synaptic connections it received for ones now appropriate for the muscle it happened to innervate (Weiss, 1950). Recent work has given evidence for the opposite view, that motor nerves of lower vertebrates reconnect with their correct muscles, even when surgically diverted into foreign muscles or strange parts of the limb (Mark 1965, 1969).

Detailed analysis of the recovery of movement of fish eye muscles and salamander limb muscles, after section and regeneration of the motor nerves that supply them, has shown why Weiss was misled. In the case of the eye, foreign nerve fibres, forced into a muscle, the nerve supply of which had been previously removed, would form functional synaptic neuromuscular functions which took command of the muscle and produced reversed reflex eye movements, much as would Sperry's reversal of the sensory component of reflex mechanisms. When the correct innervation grew back into the cross-innervated muscle the reversed reflexes disappeared as soon as the correct movements returned (Marrotte and Mark, 1970a). Subsequent electronmicroscopic examination of the muscles revealed two nerve supplies, both of which terminated in morphologically normal neuromuscular junctions (Marotte and Mark, 1970b; Mark, Marotte, and Mart, 1972). All the behavioural evidence, backed up by electrophysiological recordings and measurement of muscle contraction, however, pointed to the fact that while both sets of nerves brought impulses down to the muscle, with the timing appropriate for those motoneurones, synaptic transmission and muscle contraction only occurred in response to impulses from the original mononeurones (Mark and Marotte, 1972).

It is not necessary any more to single out neuromuscular connection formation. The mechanisms are the same as those in other systems. Each muscle is somehow marked in a way that makes it recognizable by sprouts of motoneurone axon. The correct innervation pattern depends upon a set of embryologically marked motoneurones developing functional connections with the set of similarly marked muscles. Physiological, rather than anatomical, connectivity restores the connection pattern.

Chemospecificity of neurones

Most of the early evidence for what Sperry (1963) has now called chemospecificity in the development of neuronal connections, has come from experiments like those described above on lower vertebrates, fish, (Attardi and Sperry, 1963), newts (Cronly-Dillon, 1968), and frogs (Maturana, Lettvin, McCulloch, and Pitts, 1959; Gaze, 1960). They were good for this because their embryology was well known and the powers of regeneration of the nervous system enormous. Higher vertebrates do not regrow optic nerves and show much less flexibility in neuromuscular repair. However, there is not any good reason for thinking that such refined developmental mechanisms do not apply equally to the embryogenesis of more complicated nervous systems and no other theory challenges this one at the moment (Sperry, 1963).

The development of chemospecificity in retinal and optic lobe neurones has been studied since the 1950s by doing the eye rotation experiment earlier and earlier in larval development. There comes a stage at which the operation does not result in reversed vision in the adult. This is very early in development, at about embryological stage twenty-six in certain frog tadpoles when the retina is only about twenty cells across (Jacobson, 1968a). The time of specification coincides with a sudden reduction in the rate of DNA synthesis in the retina but there is no information as to what else happens in the retina at that time(Jacobson, 1968b). Specification follows a timetable with the anteroposterior axis becoming fixed before the dorsoventral (Stone, 1944; Szekely, 1954a). Presumably morphogenetic substances produced by the surrounding epidermis set up diffusion gradients at right angles and some derivative of this gradient becomes a fixed part of the retinal cell's heritage (Grafstein and Burgen, 1964). This idea of morphogenetic gradients is common in embryology even though the physical nature of the gradient in unknown (Child, 1941).

The retina grows tremendously after the stage of cytochemical specification, by adding on cells at the circumference but the gradient of specificities is maintained through this growth. The fact that connection-specifying markers grow with an organ suggests that the rank order of cells across the original line of the gradient is what is signalled, rather than the precise individual location in the sequence. The development of the tadpole visual system provides a fascinating example of this. Whereas the retina grows circumferentially, the optic lobe to which the axons of the retinal cells project grows mainly from its posterior and medial margins. Yet, whenever the retino-rectal projections are mapped by electrophysiological methods, during development, the whole of the visual field occupies the whole of the tectum (Gaze, Chung, and Keating, 1972). Normally the temporal, or posterior, side of the retina projects to the front of the tectum. As new temporal ganglion cells develop and send their axons into the tectum they must come to occupy synaptic sites at the most anterior end of this structure, sites already in possession of an innervation by the previously most temporal retinal axons. All the functional connections formed all the way across the tectum must therefore shift down so the rank order is still respected and the projection complete (Fig. 6). It is not known whether the shift of connections involves the growth of new synapses or whether it is a change in the efficacy of widespread synapses formed during the initial ingrowth of retinal axons. The end result is that the whole of the growing visual system remains in charge of the motor system, and whether for defence or for the finding of food, the function of visuomotor location is crucial to developing free-swimming larvae.

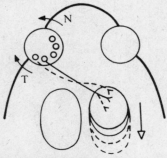

FIG. 6. Growth of the eye and tectum. Cells added by circumferential growth of the retina on the temporal side always project to the anterior tectum. Since this is now growing too, new connections must displace previous ones down towards the growing posterior margin of the optic tectum. (After Gaze, Chung, and Keating, 1972.)

Other experimental manipulations of chemospecific reconnections show topographical rank order to be respected, rather than a precise fixed point to point correspondence. If the eyes from two embryo toads are removed and cut in two in the dorso-ventral axis, two halves from each eye may be pressed together to make a single composite eye (Szekely, 1954b). If the two halves are both from the anterior or posterior half of the original, one can make a composite eye that has two front halves (nasal retinae, or two back halves, temporal retinae). Normally cells from each half retina only project to half of the tectum anterior or posterior. When the cells from compound eyes grow out to the brain each half spreads its projection over the whole of the tectum. Since each half eye is a mirror image of the other and each looks out to half the visual field, electrophysiological mapping of the system shows that any one spot on the tectum may be excited from two symmetrical loci in opposite halves of visual space (Gaze, Jacobson, and Szekely, 1963, 1965). There is no vacant optic lobe corresponding to the missing half retina (Fig. 7). Optic axons fill it up in topological order and do not leave gaps.

Rank order is also shown to govern reconnection of optic nerve fibres to fish optic lobes when a proportion of the optic lobe is removed (Gaze and Sharma, 1970; Yoon, 1971 (Fig. 7); Yoon, 1972). All the optic fibres compress themselves into the remaining area of tectum, keeping their order the same but

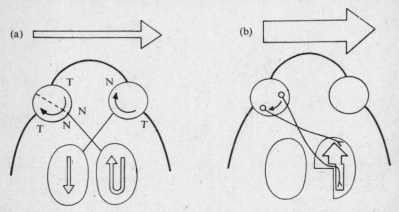

FIG. 7. Two experiments suggesting that retino-tectal connections are made according to rank order rather than precise cell to cell correspondences. (*a*) Connections formed by compound double temporal eyes. The compound eyes are made early in development by pressing together two half-eyes taken from donor animals and replacing one original eye of the host with the composite. When connections to the tectum form, each temporal half retina spreads its projection over the whole tectum so that each spot on the optic lobe is excited from two points in the visual field and there are no vacant areas of tectum. (After Gaze, Jacobson, and Szekely, 1963.) (*b*) Excision of the caudio-medial segment of one tectum. The projections from the eye to the missing area are compressed over into the remaining quadrant. The whole visual field is once again projected on to the tectum although the projection to the posterior tectum is compressed relative to that of the anterior tectum. (After Yoon, 1971.)

spreading over only part of the original space. The synaptic mechanism of this spreading or compression of projection from one set of neurones to another is not yet known.

THE FUNCTION OF EMBRYOLOGICALLY DETERMINED NERVE CIRCUITS

Nothing is more misleading from the developmental viewpoint than to consider the brain primarily as the organ of the mind. In animal evolution the brain emerges at the front end of a primitive nervous system as a control system linking the distance receptors, eyes, ears, and chemical senses, to certain well-defined motor patterns, which are essential for very existence. Most of the examples taken refer to the mechanism for location of objects of possible significance in the map of the visual space surrounding the animals, that is generated in the brain according to nerve-impulse activity in the central projections of the mosaic of light receptor units in the eye. This is a space code in the sense used in Chapter 1, which on passing into the optic lobe emerges as a pattern of muscle action that leads to movement towards the appropriate part of the visual world. By far the bulk of the nervous system is given over to these organized patterns of activity. So important is this aspect on inherited behaviour that embryological mechanisms of great precision and power ensure that the basic patterns do develop in each individual, no matter what the circumstances of its own development.

The repair of nerve connections to peripheral mammalian ganglia of the autonomic system shows evidence of the same process of precise matching of preganglionic motoneurones to ganglion cells (Langley, 1895; Murray and Thompson, 1957; Guth and Bernstein, 1961; Landmesser and Pilar, 1970). The same laws appear to govern the formation of nervous connections in invertebrates; to cricket legs (Sahota and Edwards, 1969), or sensory cells (Edwards and Palka, 1971), the fly's eye (Horridge and Meinertzhagen, 1970), and interneurones connecting segmental ganglia in the leech (Baylor and Nicholls, 1971; Jansen and Nicholls, 1972).

Cellular diversity is the key to the rigid inheritance of these behavioural patterns, diversity of shape, biochemical characteristics and of connectivity of neurones. All of these are produced by the operation of genetic and developmental mechanisms, mainly outside the influence of experience or the presence of absence of impulse activity in the component cells. Such mechanisms impose coarse and fine structure upon the brain so that inherited behaviour with its critical role in survival emerges willy-nilly as the background upon which each individual animal begins its own existence, with environmental and social contingencies that now become a matter for individual adaptability.

In answer to the questions posed at the beginning of the chapter, it is easier to believe, at least until it is proven otherwise, that the framework of individual behaviour is inherited and specified by embryological mechanisms unaffected by individual experience. By and large we behave as do the rest of our species and individual variations in behaviour are small in relation to the inherited differences in behaviour that separate different kinds of animals. Such predictability of the behaviour of a species has come to be recognized as having a critical role in speciation and evolution, and in the main there is no reason to distinguish the mechanisms of behavioural inheritance and expression from those of other inherited characteristics. Precious little variation is allowed, and the genetic mechanisms guard the development of behaviour from direct environmental pressures as effectively as for any other phenotypic character.

One must ask again whether the principles that sound reasonable for the automatic behaviour of lower animals could apply to man with his immense learning ability and added facility of language as a means of maintaining social evolution. I rather think they can, and that the view of the brain as a blank slate for eduction, in the form mainly of verbal learning, is a biased one that does not take into account the already highly restricted nature of learnable material. As a visitor from another world, or a member of another species on this one, an observer would notice first the similarities in the verbal expressions of man before he noticed differences, universal use of the larynx and muscles of respiration, similar vowel sounds interrupted by consonants imposed by intricate co-ordination patterns of the mouth, lips, and tongue, the temporal sequence of sounds broken into words and phrases of similar length, and so on. Also the development of language in young children goes through a highly predictable pattern, with the timetable and early sounds being unaffected by culture or language. Obviously there is a rigidly programmed development of audio-motor co-ordination that unfolds the raw material for a communication system at about the same speed and in the same manner irrespective of parental or cultural pressures (Lenneberg, 1967).

This amount of developmental biological order generates

as much wonder as to its informational requirements as do the refined mechanisms that can attach a social meaning to any sequence of sounds. And yet even here the detailed analysis of grammar has shown surprising similarities between languages that are apparently unrelated in their origins or verbal components. Only certain symbolic patterns are available to the human brain. The fine structure of language, the precise symbols adopted within the physiological limits, and the precise attachment of meaning to such symbols are less impressive than the similarities of the physiology of language (Chomsky, 1967).

If one accepts this attitude to the brain and extends it to its highest functions, language, and other symbolic means of social communications, there are important repercussions for possible mechanisms of learning. It ceases to be a matter of depositing in a featureless memory bank all those events of possible adaptive significance. Learning becomes a matter of comparatively minute adjustments of inherited and genetically determined behaviour patterns, in accordance with individual experience.

Learning only happens, in fact is only worth it, in the biological sense, in association with inherited behaviour of proven adaptive power. Therefore, far from looking in the brain for a set of uncommitted nerve cells that are only to record life's experiences, we should direct attention to parts of the brain that have proven so successful that their inheritance is worth a massive investment of genetic material. These are aspects of behaviour that are likely to benefit from a small individual influence that will further enhance their present effectiveness. Similarly, at the cellular level, the mechanism of learning is best sought in the mechanisms of behavioural inheritance, with known links to the morphogenesis of the brain, adapted in some way to exert a small but obviously significant pressure on the development or maintenance of such brain networks according to individual experience.

4 · *Experiments on Memory*

IN order to try and find out what happens in the brain during the formation of memories there are two main experimental strategies. One may measure as precisely as possible certain aspects of brain function during the process of memory making and try and detect a change that matches perfectly in timing and in intensity the emergence of a behavioural memory. Or one may consider the likely possibilities and by the use of progressively refined physical or chemical treatments to the brain during the time of memory formation, seek to interrupt the process. A list of all the known means of interruption or inhibition of memory plus a knowledge of how such treatments affect nerve cells and their metabolism should eventually allow the probable metabolic sequences of memory to be pieced together.

These two strategies are common to many attempts at the scientific analysis of complicated matters that are initially beyond the competence of ordinary observation and ordinary mathematical description. A good parallel comes from the history of early observation on the cause and treatment of infectious disease at the end of last century. Most of the real advances in physical medicine stemmed directly from discoveries made at this time, even antibiotics and the techniques of transplantation surgery. Scientific knowledge of memory is now in a state that corresponds to bacteriology and microbial pathogenesis a hundred years ago.

At this time two German scientists with special but divergent abilities led the search for the understanding of the catastrophic diseases, Robert Koch and Paul Erlich (Sourkes, 1967). The idea of infection in transmission of disease was familiar from centuries of observation. What was lacking was a clue as to the nature of the agent, the mechanism of infection, and what to do about it.

Koch (1880) studied the microbial concomitants of infection and by usual laboratory skill, in the course of which he invented many of the bacteriological techniques used today, solid culture media, staining, and photomicrography, succeeded in isolating the bacteria causing anthrax, tuberculosis, and cholera. In setting up the proof of the crucial pathogenic role of his isolated organisms he made use of the following postulates, which he derived from his teacher, Henle, many years before:

(1). The organism must be found in all cases of the disease and its distribution in the body should be in accordance with the lesions observed.
(2). The organism should be cultivated outside the body in pure culture for several generations.
(3). The isolated organism should reproduce the disease in other susceptible animals.

On satisfaction of the third postulate of course, one had to go back to the first, the second, and come up to the third again.

Erlich (1956) on the other hand, did not stem from the great bacteriological schools but was a gifted organic and synthetic chemist who was also educated in medicine. His interest was awakened by the unequal reaction of the body tissues to staining dye-stuffs, which he interpreted as evidence of chemical differences in the structure and metabolism of body cells. He never lost his preoccupation with the differential chemical affinities of living cells. This, coupled with his ability to think in chemical structural terms that could conjure up the likely configuration of reactive sites on cells, led to the development in his hands of many histochemical methods of use in other biological sciences and also to theoretical and practical work on antibodies, immunity, cancer, and antibacterial chemo-

therapy. The two men were not independent. Koch used
Erlich's method of differential staining of tubercle bacilli in
identifying the causal organism of tuberculosis; Erlich's observations on differential sensitivity of micro-organisms and
cells led to the development of arsenical compounds as the
first effect antimicrobial treatment for syphilis and yaws,
which soon led to the sulphonamides for other bacterial
diseases.

The analogy with memory is important. Koch's method was
to follow the natural process by skilful techniques to isolate
the factors which paralleled the course of the disease, and then
by rigorous methods prove their unique capabilities in its
reproduction. Erlich's method was to try and imagine, on the
basis of a deep knowledge of structural chemistry and the
reactions of living things, how different tissues might be expected to react with molecules of known configuration, and
how such differential reactions could be used to inhibit specifically the ill results of disease, either by toxic effect on the
bacteria or encouraging the defence of the unwilling host
animal.

This is all we can do for memory, look for metabolic or
structural parallels, or, preferably on the basis of the available
neurophysiological insight, try to devise specific inhibitors,
the nature of which will illuminate the normal process.

*Biological concomitants of memory and the problem of
control experiments*

It is easier to begin with Koch's approach because it has
yielded nothing until very recently and the current work is a
long way from satisfying the neurological equivalents of Koch's
postulates. The method is almost bound to fail to show the
critical events needed for memory because, normally, animals
or men never stop making memories. One can take the view
that all acquisition of information is memory, even though
the use of the information may not be apparent until later.
No matter how behavioural situation is set up no amount
of environmental manipulation can prohibit memory formation.

On the other hand it is easy nowadays to think up a situation
in which behavioural change can be made to be dependent

upon memories formed in relation to a known sensory stimulus or motor act, as explained in Chapter 2. Therefore measurement of neural concomitants of such change are theoretically possible, assuming one knew what to try and measure. These experiments need as a rule quite strong sensory stimuli (electric shocks of punishing intensity are commonly used) and the learning requires a change in bodily activity, either more or less to make itself apparent. All of these events could produce nervous changes independent of their contribution to memory.

The way out of this difficulty is to pair experimental animals with others that receive identical stimuli, as near as possible, but with the time relations between them so arranged that no permanent behavioural change becomes associated with the stimulus that serves as a basis for memory formation in the experimental animal. For example, in a Pavlovian conditioning experiment the conditioned stimulus is usually an innocuous one such as a quiet sound or moderate flash of light which is always followed at a fixed short interval by the unconditional stimulus, the usually stronger and often unpleasant stimulus that produces the unconditioned response, such as flexion of the leg in response to shock to the foot. Conditioning occurs when the innocuous stimulus begins to produce leg flexion, the conditioned response. Paired control animals may be given the conditioned and unconditioned stimuli in any order and time interval (non-contingent foot shock), and conditioning in relation to the chosen conditioned stimulus will not occur.

It is true that under these circumstances there is no learning of a new response in connection with a defined stimulus, but who is to say there is no learning at all (Krech, 1972). No matter what the technique for delivery of the non-contingent stimuli, confinement in the test apparatus, with all these various stimuli and no simple behavioural recourse allowed, is likely to be even more stressful to the experimental animal than a successful conditioning experiment. Cascades of memories may be made in relation to each punishing event and all that is lacking is their attachment to a chosen arbitrary sensory stimulus.

If it was known just where in the brain the physiological

events following this chosen sensory stimulus became converted into the raw material of memory, one might be able to find out about the transformation by study of the concomitants. But we do not know where to look. The problem in these experiments is to separate, in the brain, the memories made in relation to a known sensory event in the experimental animals, from memories made in relation to an unknown number of unknown sensory stimuli in the control animals. In principle this is harder than trying to find a memory in a brain that is known to contain one, in comparison to one that is known not to.

The only way to stop memories from forming is to prevent or greatly reduce sensory input. This is not a suitable control because one cannot distinguish, in the experimental case, the consequences of sensory stimulation from those subsequent neurological events likely to be concerned specifically in memory formation (Bateson, 1970). A hopeless outlook either way, at least in the search for the unique mechanism of memory.

GAINS IN KNOWLEDGE WITH KOCH'S APPROACH
Anatomical

However, it is useful to know how behavioural complexes, environmental stimuli, adaptive behaviour and general activity do affect the structure, physiology, and bio-chemistry of the brain, specially if there has been engineered a behavioural change in relation to a particular environmental stimulus. It is reasonably certain that environmental impoverishment in rats is associated with a slight but reliable reduction in thickness of the cerebral cortex. Branching of neurone cell processes appears to be less extensive and the meshwork of fine fibres and process that separate nerve cell bodies in the cortex is not as extensive (Rosenzweig, Bennet, and Diamond, 1972). Biochemical measurements also show differences, and the behavioural adaptability, as measured by maze learning and other tests, is also inferior (Krech, Rozenzweig, and Bennet, 1960). These effects are produced over a long time. The mechanism is unknown. It occurs in rodents which are unusual in growing continuously over their lifetime and it may be related to hormonal changes induced by environmental manipulation (Walsh, Budtz-Olsen, Penney, and

Cummins 1969). Anatomical changes in association with a specific learning situation have not been discovered.

Physiological. There are very many accounts of changes in the electrical activity of the brain in learning, some of which are even large enough to be recorded by sensitive electronic instruments outside the human skull. They range from modulation of frequency of evoked responses to rhythmic stimuli in some brain regions (Morrell 1961; John, 1967; Elazar and Adey, 1967), and changes in time relations of naturally occurring rhythmic activities of different parts of the cerebral cortex, to detailed observations on the firing frequency and pattern of single neurons (Olds and Hirano, 1969). There is absolutely no doubt that when the behaviour of an animal swings towards special dependence upon an experimentally chosen sensory stimulus the neuronal response to this stimulus changes. The changes do not occur everywhere in the brain, and by complex and difficult experiments involving the recording of the electrical discharges of neurones in all parts of the brain during conditioning experiments, a picture of the changing patterns should slowly build up (Olds, Disterhoff, Segal, Kornblith, and Hirsh, 1972).

These experiments do not help in answering the central question because they are about learning and not about memory. They are an attempt to describe the way in which the fleeting patterns of brain activity profit from memories formed to move into new configurations allowing behavioural acts to emerge from changing sensory states. Pursued simply as mapping experiments in space and time they are unsuited to discovering which nerve cells have had the fundamental changes and which are engaged in erecting the neuronal pattern for planned behaviour on the basis of the changes.

On the analogy with infectious disease these experiments correspond to describing the distribution, and pathological consequences of the body's reaction, to an invading organism. They do not show which changes are uniquely dependent on the presence of the infecting organism and, of course, give no ideas about the real nature of the bacterium.

Biochemical. The development of micromethods for protein

and RNA analysis has enabled similar experiments to be done on biochemical correlates of neuronal use and perhaps learning. Since 1943, H. Hyden has studied the changes in nucleic acid and protein composition of stimulated neurones. Normal physiological use of neurones has been shown to cause an increase in the amount and a change in the base ratios of extracted RNA. This occurs in neurones associated with the maintenance of balance during a task that required rats to learn to climb a tight-rope (Hyden and Egyházi, 1962), and also in neurones of the cerebral cortex in a task that required the transfer of handedness in a manipulative task (Hyden and Egyházi, 1964).

Unusual technical skill and patience are required for these experiments because owing to the cellular variety of the brain only estimates made on single neurones are really useful. Therefore each nerve cell has to be dissected out individually by micromanipulation and then the chemical methods used must detect and analyse less than 10^{-8}g of nucleic acid or protein (Hyden and Lange, 1968). Such experiments have demonstrated the tight link between impulse activity and RNA synthesis. In fact, neurones have no rival as producers of RNA and new protein and this synthetic metabolism is clearly bound to the electrical activity of the membrane. There must be something in this that is relevant to memory but so far the connection is not established. Further clues come from experiments in which an acidic protein rich in glutamic acid and occurring largely in glial cells in the brain was measured and found to be increased in amount in cortical cells in the transfer of handedness experiments, only on one side of the brain, corresponding to the hand used (Hyden and Lange, 1970). Antibodies made against this protein and applied directly to the brain prevent the acquisition of the handedness transfer.

These are fascinating and admirable experiments but so far have told us nothing about memory beyond to emphasize the unbreakable ties between the manufacture of neuronal protein and the events of electrical signalling. Even the block of acquired behaviour by antibrain antibodies merely indicates that perhaps new learning is more susceptible to disruption by immunological attack of the brain than are older learned responses or instinctive behaviour. The experiments are not transferable to just any behavioural situation. No similar biochemical findings can be correlated with rats learning to run a maze for example (a correspondent, 1972). So this work has not yet led us closer to real understanding of memory.

Other workers have pursued this path of research without the use of ultramicromethods of biochemical analysis by using particularly strong behavioural methods. One of the most stable kinds of learning is that of some newly hatched birds, which develop behavioural bonds to their parents at a critical period in the first few days of their life. This is known as imprinting because the bond formed is lifelong, more or less irreversible and directs the subsequent social and sexual behaviour of the individual (Slukin, 1965). Imprinting is associated with an increase in RNA, synthesis in the visual areas of the chicken brain (Bateson, Horn, and Rose, 1972). The new RNA may be linked to learning or to the reception of the appropriate visual stimuli. It has not yet been possible to differentiate between these hypotheses because many visual stimuli result in imprinting. Imprinting may only be prevented by using different, less behaviourally effective visual stimuli, which of course will have different sensory consequences in the brain from those of the effective stimuli.

Other attempts have been made to find biochemical correlates of learning by taking particular care with behavioural control groups during avoidance conditioning (Adair, Wilson, and Glassman, 1968). These experiments have shown an increase in RNA synthesis under certain behavioural conditions but as far as the contribution of learning to this increased synthesis they are subject to the same criticism as the work on imprinting.

One of the most delicate techniques of molecular biology, competitive hybridization of RNA strands, has been used to try and detect new RNA made in the brain during learning. It has been briefly reported to suceed (Machlus and Gaito, 1967), and fail (Von Hungen, 1971).

Could there be a memory virus? Many people have had the

idea that the protein made in the brain may have some very direct connection with behavioural memory (Katz and Halstead, 1950; Booth, 1967; Glassman, 1969; Gaito, 1971). After all, instinctive behaviour depends upon precisely controlled neuronal development under gene control, why should not acquired behaviour share a close association with stable genetic molecules. If this were so it is conceivable that each behavioural memory might have a direct molecular counterpart in a characteristic protein, specified by a characteristic messenger RNA. It is the theory of the memory virus, having a recognizable existence outside the brain and being capable of reorganizing brain function so as to read out, in behaviour, its own encoded message. Very many attempts have been made to prove the existence of a transmissible element of memory, by experiments that are analogous to those which proved the unique importance of pathogenic bacteria in disease.

Some of these have worked and some have not. The great difficulties are in the behavioural techniques that experimenters are forced to use to reveal the presence of memory. Behavioural change of course depends upon many things other than memory: hunger, thirst, fatigue, hormonal state, generalized reactions to toxic substances cover some of the internal variables, familiarity or strangeness of the environment, appropriateness of the task for the species used, social interactions with other animals, either directly or by sounds or characteristic odour, represent some of the external factors. The relative weights of these contributions to behaviour vary with species, strain, age, method of raising animals, and so on. One can only imagine the complexity of a behavioural experiment that controlled adequately for all these matters and revealed the crucial dependence of a behavioural act on a complex memory reflecting a delicate perceptual distinction. Most behavioural methods have been fairly crude, such as avoidance of the dark for a lighted compartment, or inhibition of a tendency to move from a small platform or ledge on to the floor. Most commonly the animals were rats and mice. The experiments therefore have consisted of training animals in such a task, usually by punishment for errors, extracting the brain for likely molecules, RNA protein or polypeptides, and injecting the extract, with suitable control groups, into

a new population that are tested for performance of the same
task (Reinis, 1965; Ungar and Oceguera-Navarro, 1965;
Babich, Jacobson, Bubash, and Jacobson, 1965; Fjerdingstad,
1969).

It is remarkable that very often these experiments do work
and a proportion of the recipient animals show a fragment of
behaviour reminiscent of that of the donor. Why is this so?
Does this prove that memory molecules do exist and they may
reprogramme the recipient brains? In most cases the conclusions must lead to a refutation of this hypothesis or a guarded
acceptance of the experimental facts, but not of any easily testable hypothesis (Brindley, 1970). A good control is to test the
effect of donation of extracts of other organs, the liver for
example, which has been shown on occasions to be as effective
as brain (Frank, Stein, and Rosen, 1970), supporting the idea
of transferable behaviour but not the idea of the transfer of
specific information related to brain function in memory. In
other situations transmissible behaviour is reported to come
only from brain extracts. Further checks to the acceptance of
the implications of these experiments has come from the extraction procedures, which have usually been crude, and the
route of access of the extract to the brain. Effective behavioural
changes may be produced by intraperitoneal injection of extract but very little or none of the larger molecules injected
may ever reach the brain. Moreover, the experiments are
difficult to replicate from one laboratory to another (Byrne
et al., 1966), which is not necessarily a criticism of technique
but does emphasize that the effects are often marginal changes
in behaviour, in spite of giving results of statistical significance, and they may be completely masked or even inverted by
some of the previously mentioned non-specific effects.

One candidate as a molecular carrier of behaviour is a poly-
peptide produced in the brains of animals trained to avoid the
dark, which has been analysed and synthesized and then shown
to have the same transfer effects as the original brain extract
(Ungar, Desiderio, and Parr, 1972; and see also Stewart, 1972).
If these claims can be substantiated it sounds as though they
come close to Koch's postulates for the identification of a
transmitting agent. Would this be a finding of equal importance to the discovery of the tubercle bacillus? I think not, at

this stage of brain science, mainly because it illuminates nothing else about the known workings of the brain. What is needed is a molecular explanation for acquired behaviour where each step in the process can be understood in terms of anatomy, physiology, or biochemistry of brain cells.

Nothing startling comes from the finding that a chemical compound can induce similar behaviour in recipient animals. The effects of many hormones and drugs such as narcotics, alcohol and cerebral stimulants like amphetamine, are to produce behavioural changes which, in a tightly controlled situation can bias the actions of all animals in the same direction. No one would consider these effects as a specific chemical transfer of behaviour. Should a conditioned brain, responding to a certain stimulus, manufacture an excess of a certain metabolic product which can be made to produce biased behaviour in other animals, one should not be too surprised. Neither the origin of the potent molecules nor the behavioural change can be related unequivocally to the formation of effective memory (Dyal, 1971).

Biochemical methods applied to the extraction of a single kind of molecule from the whole brain are too remote from the intimate chemical mechanisms that must exist for maintaining the fantastic cellular individuality of the brain. Behavioural methods measuring a single reaction of complicated mammals are too remote from the nuances of perceptual distinction that go to make up the raw material, we know, of human memories. It would be imprudent to deny that chemically transmissible behaviour exists. One has the uneasy feeling from all this literature, contradictory and incomplete as it is, that something is there (Byrne, 1970; Ungar, 1970; Gaito, 1972). The question is whether this represents a mainstream of memory research or whether the lack of coherence of these experiments with the other brain disciplines rules out scientific progress along these lines.

Some years ago great hopes were held that a short-cut to the chemical treatment of cancer might come from a massive research programme into natural biological chemicals from plants and animals, which could be tested quite arbitrarily for their effectiveness against tumours of laboratory animals. Nothing has come of it. Effective molecular anti-cancer treatment, such as it is, has come from intelligent application of basic discoveries of molecular biology and cellular immunology. Similarly with memory. Good understanding can only grow out of soundly based fundamental biological knowledge. Nowadays even if we somehow knew for certain the exact molecular constitution of a real memory molecule, one doubts the ability of current biochemical techniques to recognize it in the brain, along with all the other metabolic products of normal brain function. One doubts also the sensitivity of known behavioural methods to reveal the induction of one discrete memory, among the enormous number of individual behaviour patterns of an animal with any experience at all of individual existence.

The most telling criticism of chemical memory transfer experiments is not to deny the possibility of the effects, or to denigrate the investigators, but to say they are before their time. This is just as serious a scientific criticism as to say the work is old-fashioned and repetitive. It means that even if such research stumbled upon something of real significance, which perhaps it already has, it is unlikely that adequate standards of proof could be attained to satisfy the rest of the scientific community and the finding could not be exploited because of the surrounding chasms of ignorance as to other aspects of brain function.

It is the claim of researchers in this field that their findings could illuminate the other areas. Neither neurophysiology nor neuroembryology at the moment appears to be in a state to assimilate a finding of the precision and refinement appropriate for a molecular code for memory.

INHIBITION OF MEMORY FORMATION

But what of Erlich's approach, the discovery of the normal through knowledge of specific inhibitors. Here the outlook is decidedly more open. In principle, one could find out the anatomical location of memory, and the physiological and biochemical steps for its registration by a combination of discrete spatial damage to the brain and specific inhibition of metabolic pathways.

Anatomical

The anatomical work came first, growing naturally out of the discoveries of the separate location of various functions of the brain about a hundred years ago. From localized destruction, deliberate or by disease, paroxysmal stimulation by epileptic discharges or by well-controlled electrical stimulation it emerged that certain aspects of behaviour sensation and motor powers were specially related to certain parts of the brain. Experiments on the involvement of brain areas in memory were done in the 1930s by Karl Lashley (1950, 1960) who spent most of his scientific life in search of what he popularised as the engram, the word he adopted for the physical record of memory. The method was to train rats on various tasks, such as visual discrimination and maze learning and estimate the deficit in performance caused by damage to the brain, mainly the cerebral cortex. His conclusion was that the deficits such gross damage produced were proportional to the total area of cortex eliminated not to the precise location.

This was an unexpected finding at the time when much other neurological research emphasized the topographical features of brain organization and the sensory and motor maps produced by space-coded neuronal systems were being discovered and rediscovered in greater and greater detail. But Lashley was a good experimenter, with a great deal of insight into mechanisms of behaviour and a much more realistic appreciation of the brain than most physiologists of the time and his general conclusions have stood up well. Localization of function for memories governing the behaviour of the whole animal in its spatial environment is not precise. The cortex is more or less equipotential in this respect and similar levels of performance can be sustained by a brain with equivalent amounts of damage in different areas.

This conclusion is about the ability of the whole animal to behave in an appropriate way and gives no clue as to the neurological strategy of behaviour. Massive deficits in primarily visual areas could be compensated for by shifting the perceptual load for analysing the environment on to olfactory or tactile senses or by simplifying the visual perceptions required, more emphasis on overall colour and brightness and less on detailed pattern recognition.

The sensible conclusion from Lashley's eminently sensible work is not that memories are somehow broadcast into the brain in a fragmented form in which each brain region contains only a trace of the message but that memories for behaviour are made at a level of organization in the brain where simultaneous analysis of the maximum amount of converging sensory information becomes possible, that is where integration of visual, tactile, auditory, olfactory, and other sensations all contribute to selection of the most useful motor patterns. Such organization is by nature distributed among the neurones connected to the appropriate space-coded maps and a certain amount of equivalence or redundancy in the neuronal circuits collecting this information is to be expected. It is not incompatible in the slightest with changes, perhaps minute ones, at certain anatomically recognizable nerve cells or synapses being the physical memory.

More recent research of the same nature has begun to show more specific defects in learned behaviour from localized brain damage, but none of this is on a fine enough scale to point out which nerve cells might store memory and of course it cannot reveal how they might do it. These experiments can contribute to an understanding of overall brain function involved in memory and one fascinating finding has come from observation mainly of clinical cases in which bilateral damage to some of the phylogenetically older parts of the cerebral cortex results in a permanent defect in the ability to form new memories (Milner and Penfield, 1955). The retention of old ones is less affected. These areas, the hippocampus and limbic forebrain in anatomical terms, therefore seem to be somehow concerned with the organization of brain function for induction of memory in regulating mechanisms of selective spatial attention or short-term memory (Olds, 1972). The study of the neurophysiology of the hippocampal cortex is a matter of great importance for memory research and is technically not too difficult (Lømo, 1971). However, once again this does not relate directly to the most fundamental question in the physiology of memory, the physical nature of the store, because all the neuropsychological evidence adds up to the conclusion that in spite of its transient importance in actual learning the permanent store is not located in this region. Rather, the co-operation of the hippocampal cortex is required for the easy induction of memory changes elsewhere in the brain, probably mainly in relation to neurones of the cerebral cortex.

The anatomical approach has also been tried with invertebrates. In some animals their sense organs and perceptual systems are so different from the human that knowledge of the detailed functioning of such a nervous system would have mainly local interest. An exception comes from the mollusc *Octopus vulgaris* which although remote from the vertebrates in most ways has developed an eye with a retina and lens quite analogous to man. Further investigation of the visual behaviour of octopus has shown that they have a most flexible memory system in association with vision, which allows them to profit from past experience in deciding whether to come out from their normal hiding-place and attack an object as possible food. The advantage for experimental work on memory was that the invertebrate nervous system is laid out quite differently from the vertebrate, although the nerve cells are basically the same, and it was open to a new analysis of the function of its components by observing the behavioural effect of localized damage or removal of parts of the brain. In the last forty years Young (1966) carried out research on the location of memory and the function of ancillary nervous mechanisms mediating reinforcement and the access to memory. Evidence is presented that the store of information is actually in the optic lobes, close to the mechanisms of visual perception; and various mixing, amplifying, and biasing functions necessary for the use of stored information are handled in the higher centres. Similar sub-systems serve touch learning.

This is anatomical work of the kind most relevant to physiology. It aims to discover how the conformation of nerve cells and their connections are specialized in those areas of brain more specifically related to the behavioural expression of memory. Because of its functional setting this kind of knowledge should, and often does, throw up good physiological ideas. One of the most useful, repeatedly emphasized by Young (1964), is the importance of getting away from the idea of memory as a repository of information, separate in the brain from the mechanisms of perception and response. Another most important concept is that of a repressive or selective process as being important in the neurology of memory (Young, 1965). He goes even so far as to postulate an inhibitory transmitter to do this job and emphasizes the likelihood of the small Golgi Type II neurones participating in the repressive switching. Such principles, based as they are on an appreciation of learning as an evolutionary development, and compatible with the current knowledge of brain anatomy, are valuable guidelines for physiological research. Yet, in the end, they do not help very much in the analysis of the cellular mechanism of registration of memory, which must remain complementary to this. Part of the difficulty in extending the work on the octopus to physiological problems in that the octopus nervous system is not easy to manage in electrophysiological experiments.

Physiological; the time course of memory formation

The belief that there are two mechanisms of memory, a short-term mechanism responsible for holding information, shortly after receipt, and a long-term one for permanent storage, is an old one which came mainly from clinical observation of patients who had suffered some sudden trauma to the brain, usually concussion from an accident. Such people often lose their memory for events immediately before the accident (retrograde amnesia) and find it difficult to make new memories afterwards (post-traumatic amnesia). Both these deficits improve with time but there is often a permanent period of retrograde amnesia for a few seconds, minutes, or longer preceding the accident (Russell and Nathan, 1946).

It appears that sudden disruption of brain function has a differential effect upon old and new memories, the old recovering well but the new being completely eliminated. This points to a change of state of the memory with time, it first being incorporated into the functional state of the brain where it is a potent director of behaviour but is lost completely when the moment-to-moment brain function is stopped. Later on the same memory becomes converted to a form that is more resistant.

Psychologists postulated that the first stage involved the repetitive passage of nerve impulses over marked circuits in the brain and the second stage some structural change which for ever facilitated the passage of impulses over the same circuits (Hebb, 1949). There has never been any physiological evidence for or against either hypothesis. However, the idea that the physical nature of memory storage changes with time after learning has been a strong stimulus to experimental work and since the phenomenon of retrograde amnesia was brought into the laboratory many hundreds of papers have been written on the time-dependence of memory storage.

The changing nature of the physical long-term store, evidence for which came from experimental interference with the material brain, is quite separate from the idea of the changing nature of the encoding processes in memory which came from psychological experiments, mainly with man. The psychological short-term registration and recoding processes occur immediately upon the receipt of information in time that can be measured in seconds or minutes, the physiological transformation of the mechanism of storage follows this, although for the shorter intervals the times may overlap. It is unfortunate that the phychologists and the physiologists have both adopted the term short-term memory for the first stages of both processes (Barondes and Cohen, 1968). It is probably true to say that the physiological transformation from short- to long-term storage reflects a change in the material basis of the psychological long-term memory.

Almost all work on the physiological aspects of the transformation from temporary to permanent store follows the same plan. An apparently simple memory task is devised, requiring the minimum number of trials for acquisition, preferably only one, and in groups of animals brain function is disrupted at measured intervals after training by some physical or chemical insult to the brain. Electroconvulsive shock, chemical convulsants, anaesthesis, anoxia, sudden falls of temperature are some of the commonly used treatments and they all give superficially similar results (Gibbs and Mark, 1973). If the treatment is applied very soon after learning the memory is lost and on testing a day or so later, the animals behave as if they have never experienced the learning. If the treatment is delayed progressively, a greater and greater proportion of experimental animals show memory retention at subsequent test until with a delay of some minutes to hours the treatment is quite ineffective. By plotting on a graph the relative effectiveness of the amnesic treatment against time interval between learning and its administration one can build up a curve showing the growing resistance of the memory to physical disruption, the consolidation curve. Theoretically by analysis of the consolidation curve one should be able to work out some facts about the kinetics of the transformation of the memory store.

There are numerous reasons why this has not yet been possible. Firstly, the data from different experimenters are so variable, ranging from a consolidation time of seconds to several hours. The reason for this is probably that learning experiences induce various amounts of memory, depending upon the severity of the conditions and the appropriateness of the task. A very strong memory, consolidating at the same rate as a weak one will build up enough permanent storage sooner than a weak memory, even if the process goes at a constant rate. The initial memory can be thought of as a substrate for a constant rate enzymic reaction the product of which must reach a critical absolute level before being available to direct behaviour. The more substrate the quicker the absolute level is attained. Whatever the mechanism, learning strength, even if very difficult to define or measure behaviourally, appears to affect behavioural consolidation rate (Cherkin, 1966).

This matter is not the real difficulty. Each kind of amnesic treatment, electroconvulsive shock, chemical agents, and so on will itself produce direct effects on behaviour and learning in relation to its application. Adequate experimental controls for these effects may be very difficult to obtain. For example, simple learning tasks often involve withholding otherwise spontaneous behaviour in response to a warning stimulus, which is called passive avoidance learning. If one of the effects of the amnesic treatment is to produce a conditioned emotional response that results in the animal becoming immobile, and freezing is a common response of hunted animals to a situation of great danger, then freezing will be interpreted as learned avoidance and scored as memory retention. Apparently simple experiments become almost impossibly complex the further their analysis progresses. The analysis takes great behavioural skill and patience on the part of the investigators and involves the heavy investment of time and money. There is a huge backlog of published experiments on the inhibition of memory by different physical or chemical agents each one still in the need of perceptive re-evaluation of the behavioural variables. For experiments on electroconvulsive shock much of this work has been done and there are several separate explanations of why shock might suppress recently learned behaviour, only one of which is directly concerned with the hypothetical process of memory consolidation.

The best experiments one can now envisage, incorporating the maximum control of non-specific effects on behaviour would require learning in relation to a complex visual discrimination, the specificity of which could be readily tested, and the acquired behaviour should be measured by active or passive response to both punishment and positive reward. The dose and time relations of the amnesic treatment must be varied systematically in each of the behavioural situations. This is all just too much, considering that learning time must be kept to a minimum, preferably one trial, and that each experiment requires a whole set of control groups. The era of the crude consolidation experiment has therefore passed.

The aftermath of all this work taken together is that the consolidation hypothesis, that there are sequential forms of physical memory storage, has not had to be discarded. Straight after learning past experience is strong in directing behaviour but is susceptible to a series of influences any of which will prevent a permanent change. The influences range from the behavioural: a momentary distraction by presentation of further interesting stimuli; to the physiological: fatigue, hunger, hormonal state; to the pharmacological: chemical agents that alter brain function; to the pathological: surgical or chemical attack on the brain, strong electric currents, anoxia, concussion, and so on. Acquired behaviour can survive all these if they are delayed for a variable time, of the order of minutes or hours after learning. There seems to be nothing that can be done to the physical brain, compatible with its continued life, that can permanently destroy memory once the initial susceptible period is over.

Biochemical; inhibitors of permanent memory

The extraordinary durability of memories and their extraordinary longevity meant to the earlier workers that they had somehow become incorporated into brain structure, since this was all that was left untouched by the experimental attack on the engram. But since the discovery of the molecular nature of genetic material and the use of marked radioactive tracers in biochemistry it has become apparent that the stability of most of the body structure is largely an illusion. Molecules break down, are removed and resynthesized continuously, although at varying rates, in almost all the components of all tissues. Not even DNA is immune. The stability of genetic material does not result from the inherent molecular stability of these enormous double molecules but because they have developed their own repair enzymes that can chop out a damaged fragment and replace it with the correct components corresponding to the mirror strand (Watson, 1970).

It was natural, as soon as these biological discoveries were made, to relate the stability of behavioural memories to the stability of the gene and to look for chemical similarities in their mechanisms. The naturally occurring chemical warfare of the moulds, bacteria, and viruses provided the means of investigation. Simple organisms produce chemicals that interfere with growth and some of them hit directly at the genetic mechanisms or the mechanisms of transcription and protein synthesis of other, potentially rival, organisms. Penicillin, the substance that gives the common bread mould living room on substrates that are very suitable habitats for ubiquitous bacteria, was the first to be discovered and developed and myriads of others have followed.

Many of the naturally occurring microbial poisons including the genetic ones have a greater effect on bacterial metabolism than mammalian, which is the reason why they may be used to destroy selectively invading micro-organisms, in fulfilment of Erlich's hopes. Some of the others which are very potent against mammalian enzyme systems cannot be used clinically as antibacterial agents, but knowing their major biochemical sites of action, as worked out in lower organisms, they become wonderful tools for the investigation of mammalian biochemistry, including that of memory. Specificity of action of chemical inhibitors in biochemical investigation is a relative term and as more and more is demanded of an inhibitory substance in progressively more refined experiments the contaminating side effects on other metabolic systems become more and more troublesome. The longer any drug is under investigation, the more actions it turns out to have. However, the early experiments on the effect of metabolic inhibitors of protein synthesis on memory were so striking and have been reproduced so often that they must have some very direct bearing upon the cellular mechanisms involved. The effects are much the same with substances that interfere with the synthesis of RNA from the DNA template such as Actinomycin (Barondes and Jarvik, 1964; Agranoff, Davis, Casola, and Lim, 1967; Daniels, 1971).

Under the influence of these compounds, even injected directly into the brain in a quantity that will inhibit protein synthesis, as checked biochemically, by almost 100 per cent, animals may still have no difficulty in learning a new response (Agranoff, Davis, and Brink, 1966; Barondes and Cohen, 1967; Flexner and Flexner, 1968). If the retention of the response is checked over the next few hours it slowly declines, until, about two to eight hours later, depending upon the species, task, and dose, memory can have completely disappeared, at least by behavioural criteria. Various behavioural tricks can delay the disappearance of the learned response or re-evoke it shortly after its disappearance. These include a re-enactment of at least part of the initial learning such as the readministration of the punishment for error which has been shown to restore the whole learned behaviour pattern in some experiments (Barondes and Cohen, 1968; Quartermain, McEwen, and Azmitia, 1972). These refinements are not important. In a brain without protein synthesis, learned responses are initially as strong as normal but sink to inaccessibility at an enormously accelerated rate when one considers that their potential lifetime is the same as that of the animal.

Specific chemical interruption of memory is still possible if the administration of the metabolic inhibitor is delayed for some minutes after the learning experience, the exact time being set by the experimental animal and the details of the learning situation just as with electroconvulsive shock and other physical treatments producing amnesia. So as far as time relations are concerned, antimetabolites of this nature attack the mechanism of the permanent or structural store which is developing comparatively slowly after learning. In fact the rate of decline of memory in a brain, with its protein synthesis totally inhibited, should reveal the normal rate of loss of the initial form of memory (Barondes and Cohen, 1966). This has been shown to be likely to be so in experiments on memory loss in chickens pretreated with the antibiotic cycloheximide. The rate of decline of memory, may be measured by the increasing probability of forgetting in very large numbers of birds trained on a one-trial pecking avoidance task. As the dose injected directly into the brain before learning is increased a maximum rate of loss is achieved after which increasing the dose by one hundred times has no further effect (Watts and Mark, 1971). Memory loss therefore cannot, in this experiment, be due to progressively severe general toxic effects because these should become greater with higher doses, but to a specific interference with some metabolic process in the brain. The memory remaining, which is virtually full recall ten minutes after learning in this experiment must depend upon a quite separate biochemical process that is independent of recent protein synthesis for its complete expression; a clear and, for this kind of research, a well-established experimental fact, which fits well with older findings on traumatic retrograde amnesia. Memories straight after learning are quite different from memories a short time later, not necessarily in their content or availability, although these may change too, but in their physical mechanism. They are not structural or synthetic and are more susceptible to anything that will stop the electrical activity of the brain than are old memories (Roberts and Flexner, 1969; Barondes, 1970).

The physical basis of initial memory

What therefore is characteristic of the activity of nerve cells that could possibly be the physical basis of new memory? Over thirty years ago when the most obvious characteristic of nerve impulses appeared to be their extremely short duration, about a thousandth of a second, it was thought that the impulses would have to keep going, perhaps cycling round closed circuits of nerve cells, to keep the message alive while a structural change developed.

It is now known that there are accumulated consequences of rapid impulse activity in nerve cells due to the different speeds of the action-potential permeability changes and the active metabolic ion-pumping mechanisms that restore the normal ionic constitution of the cell and its immediate environment. A stream of action potentials rapidly outstrips the pumping process and can lead to the intracellular accumulation of sodium and perhaps calcium, and the extracellular accumulation of potassium. The action-potential mechanism will still continue to work even though transmembrane differences in ionic concentrations are reduced. Long periods of minutes up to perhaps half an hour may be required for the metabolic pump to re-establish the normal distribution of ions (Keynes and Ritchie, 1965; Rang and Ritchie, 1968; Kuno, Miyahara, and Weakly, 1970).

The metabolic processes are inhibited by certain naturally occurring molecules from plants. One of these, ouabain is very potent on isolated nerve membranes as an inhibitor of sodium extrusion but has little effect on the mechanism of impulse carriage (Glynn, 1964; Baylor and Nicholls, 1969; Den Hertog, and Ritchie, 1969). A direct test of this substance on early memory, using quantitative methods of memory measurement in large numbers of young chickens has shown it to be very effective in inhibiting memory as it is stored shortly after learning, specifically the form of memory resistant to antibiotics that inhibit protein synthesis. Other substances of different chemical composition but sharing the same pharmacological actions have the same effect (Watts and Mark, 1971).

This is a good experimental clue as to the possible sequence of events in formation of early labile memory. It strongly suggests that such memory depends on some electrical or metabolic consequences of a past period of intense activity and not on continued recycling of impulses by the action-potential mechanism.

Care with inhibitors

The use of biochemical blocking agents to work out metabolic pathways has been a successful technique and there seems to be no reason why it should not work well for memory too. The main difficulty is that memory that we can recognize is made best by the intact nervous system and signalled as a change in behaviour. Whereas permanent memory is as indestructible as the brain, the initiation of memories appears to be a much more fragile process, susceptible to disorganization by non-specific effects on brain function as well as by interference with its unique metabolic pathway. Therefore great pains must be taken to try and exclude such non-specific effects on memory formation, which is experimentally demanding and gives rise to reasonable criticisms of all pharmacological studies that can never be completely answered. One must be on the outlook for metabolic and hormonal changes as well as motivational effects that could modify behaviour, effects of drugs on perception and attention, the selective process of sampling environmental information and effects on levels of activity and motor performance. For many of these potential effects it is possible to design adequate behavioural control groups.

Similarly with the recognition of memory by behavioural change, even a trained animal does not behave as a meter to register new memory. It continues to respond to the totality of its environment, present and past, in ways that are not always easy to understand. The deliberate constraint of an experimental situation designed to reveal the strength of recently learned behaviour can have very strong effects of its own, which can interact in an unpredictable fashion with newly acquired responses. Some workers regard the behavioural detection of memory as simply another form of bio-assay. This is logically so, but slightly too simple a view, given the unknown variability of the unknown number of unknown factors that contribute to an experimentally defined behavioural act.

Undoubtedly more rapid progress will be made when it is possible to study learning and memory without behaviour; that is when there is a simpler more reliable assay of memory, biochemical, physiological, or anatomical. However, when knowledge of memory reaches that point we will know the answer to the central question to which this book is devoted. The experimental problems outlined above must be managed as well as possible until this stage is reached.

DO WE HAVE A THEORY OF MEMORY?

At present the only widely accepted facts on the biological basis of memory are that it is most resistant to destruction once formed and that its formation involves a change in storage mechanism from something initially dependent upon nerve impulse activity to something dependent upon the sythesis of new proteins or polypeptides. There is little knowledge of the location of the storage process, in most brains and no knowledge of its physiological or biochemical mechanism.

5 *Learning and Electrophysiological Plasticity*

OBSERVATION of memory in the whole animal and interference with brain function during learning has brought no firm and widely accepted understanding of the physiological processes required. Why not therefore examine the physiology of the brain directly and try and detect mechanisms of flexibility or plasticity in neuronal signalling that may lead back to the understanding of behaviour? It seems a good idea generally in science to try and simplify the conditions for the production of the phenomen under study: the same might be true for the physiology of memory.

THE LONG-TERM STABILITY OF SYNAPTIC TRANSMISSION

Wherever it can be studied under controlled conditions and for a long time, however, synaptic transmission has shown itself be a reliable and predictable process. Once formed and functioning the biophysical mechanisms for manufacture, storage, and release of transmitter keep up with the demands of use. Normal frequencies of action-potential activity are converted into the discrete chemical form necessary for inter-cellular communication of excitation or inhibition in the brain. Similarly the ability of the post-synaptic cell membrane to respond to the appropriate transmitter, once developed is also in the main reliable. By uptake or enzymatic breakdown secreted transmitter is removed from the receptive area fast enough to allow signalling across the synapse at a rate appropriate for the network.

Should the rate change in the long term, say in response to new environmental conditions, the rate of manufacture of transmitter by the enzymes responsible will also change so that new demands can be met (Potter, 1969). This is well exemplified in some synapses of the involuntary nervous system controlling the functions of internal organs (Mueller, Thoenen, and Axelrod, 1969). Activity provoked changes in the enzymic machinery associated with chemical synaptic transmission are often quoted as examples of flexibility or plasticity of synaptic function (Fillenz, 1972). In a way they are, but they can also be viewed as the opposite, as examples of its reliability. This intricate biochemical mechanism has been developed to read out in functional terms the interneuronal connections made by specific developmental processes. With great economy the quantitative aspects of the biochemical mechanisms are continuously adjusted to the prevailing frequency of use of the synapse, as measured mainly it appears by the frequency of impulses in the pre-synaptic nerve fibres. It is not understood yet how this control is exerted, perhaps it is by secretion in association with the chemical transmitter of certain molecules capable of regulating enzyme production, a so-called trophic substance (Black, Bloom, Hendry, and Iversen, 1971).

If such biochemical flexibility was used as a basis of memory one would require the regulatory mechanisms to break away from control by current levels of impulse activity and retain the instructions issued at some previous time so that the amount of transmitter liberated presently was that appropriate for, say, conditions of excessive use in the past. It is not out of the question that permanent changes in the overall function of a network could be permanently modified if certain synapses held to old instructions for the quantitative aspects of transmitter metabolism rather than following current demands. However, there is no positive evidence in learning experiments that this is the case and the analogous experiments on use of isolated synapses with long-term changes in average levels of activity show only appropriate changes.

Even if the biochemical regulation of transmitter release is governed by homeostatic control to keep up with functional demands this does not imply that synaptic transmission of impulses from cell to cell is a reliable one for one event. As was explained in Chapter 1, it is the rule rather than otherwise that in order to secure discharge of a post-synaptic neurone many pre-synaptic terminals must be activated within a few milliseconds of each other so as to generate a flow of sufficient synaptic current to trigger the action potential. As the number of simultaneously active pre-synaptic terminals becomes reduced so the probability of discharge becomes lessened before falling to a negligible value. The signalling between neurones of the cerebral cortex shows features that suggest that small changes in the probability of neuronal firing dependent on fluctuating pre-synaptic activity may be an important mechanism for generating changing patterns of cortical activity (Burns, 1968).

The uncertainty, however, is generated by the geometry of neuronal connectivity and by the level of activity in the connections. The synaptic process of transmitter secretion and membrane response shows great consistency, and modifiable synapses that do permanently change their effectiveness following their own impulse activity have not yet been discovered. From our current knowledge of synaptic transmission, where reliability of long-term action is the main finding, it seems hopeless to build a theory of the modifiability of brain and behaviour upon this aspect of intercellular communication alone.

SHORT-TERM CHANGES IN SYNAPTIC TRANSMISSION

The short-term modifiability of synaptic transmission on the other hand is well established and ubiquitous. At the neuromuscular junction the process of transmission of one impulse is followed by a sequence of facilitatory and inhibitory events at increasing intervals; rapid facilitation of some milliseconds duration, that appears to decline in two phases (Mallart and Martin, 1967), and then an opposing process of depression lasting some seconds or longer. Which one of these processes will dominate and extend its influence upon the control of the post-synaptic cell by the pre-synaptic terminal depends on the exact experimental conditions.

Many experiments of this kind demonstrate that the release

of transmitter in response to a nerve impulse is not independent of preceding impulses carried by the same terminal. The actual release may depend upon the fusion of transmitter-containing intracellular vesicles with the outer cell membrane and the subsequent rupture of the vesicle into the extracellular space in contact with the post-synaptic membrane. The process of release, perhaps adherence and rupture of vesicles, depends largely upon the inflow of calcium ions into the terminal from the extracellular space during the action potential (Katz and Miledi, 1965).

Two factors govern the amount of active calcium in the terminal, both of which are dependent upon the immediate past history of action potentials. Calcium is not inactivated immediately and may persist in trace amounts for long enough to accumulate when action potential frequency is high (Katz and Miledi, 1968). Secondly, if the action potential was prolonged or increased in magnitude calcium inflow per impulse would be increased. This is exactly what does happen as a result of rapidly (500 s) repeated impulse activity in any nerve fibre. Each action potential is produced by the rapid sequential inflow of sodium and outflow of potassium ions. The re-establishment of resting concentrations particularly the extrusion of sodium requires a metabolic pump, quite separate from the mechanism of the action potential and very much slower. So the passage of a high-frequency train of impulses will leave a nerve rich in sodium which is extruded over a time course of minutes. The active pumping of positive sodium ions out of the cell temporarily increases the normal internal electrical negativity of nerve cells, that is the membrane potential increases during active sodium extrusion (Rang and Ritchie, 1968). The action potential in response to stimulation takes off from a lower baseline with the result that the total potential excursion for each action potential may be both larger in amplitude and longer in time, good conditions for augmented calcium inflow and improved transmitter release. However the increased membrane potential alone is probably not the main mechanism for post-tetanic potentiation —some other aspect of the regulation of calcium ion activity in synaptic terminals probably plays a part (Gage and Hubbard, 1966).

Increased synaptic efficiency after brief high-frequency activity is a property of very many synapses studied, even those of the vertebrate neuromuscular junction where it has no apparent normal function and could scarcely be responsive to evolutionary pressures. In any neuronal network, therefore, many synapses should have this degree of modifiability. These changes however lack permanence. The maximum time for post-activity enhancement of synaptic transmission is about thirty minutes and usually times are much shorter (Lloyd, 1949).

The effect of use on nerve membrane excitability

There is another consequence of higher-frequency impulse activity of nerve cells and fibres. The same process of active sodium extrusion which temporarily increases membrane potential (hyperpolarization) has additional effects on the electrical excitability. The threshold depolarization required to initiate an action potential is a fixed fraction, about 10 per cent of the total membrane potential at any time. In normal nerve conduction the depolarizing current is provided by extracellular current flow from adjacent regions of the membrane, in synaptic transmission it comes from the synaptic current produced by chemically induced permeability changes. Whatever the mechanism, if the membrane potential is too large, the stimulating current may not be strong enough to reduce the membrane potential by an amount sufficient to start the regenerative increase of sodium permeability necessary for the action potential. This hyperpolarization block of conduction or transmission will last as long as active sodium extrusion does and will therefore also be proportional to previous impulse activity (Baylor and Nicholls, 1969). The process is very prominent and long-lasting in fine nerve fibres and small nerve cells such as make up the bulk of the brain (Ritchie and Straub, 1957).

The combined effects of short-term changes

Therefore nerve networks pointed by chemical synapses can show two opposing changes as a result of a few seconds of high-frequency electrical activity: increased transmitter effectiveness, due primarily to intracellular accumulation of calcium increasing transmitter release per impulse; and decreased electrical excitability of recently active membranes due to the hyperpolarization of cells that are in the process of active extrusion of accumulated sodium. One set of events increases transmission, the other will block it, and both have a time course of from seconds to minutes. When one considers that the simplest network may contain both excitatory and inhibitory neurones and synapses, both of which could be effected in the same way one can see that transmission through the network could either be increased by use (sensitization) or decreased by use (habituation). Many physiological preparations show these processes, some more than others, and the changes may be in either direction. These mechanisms alone, as they are now understood, cannot produce permanent changes. The self-regulatory biochemical mechanisms for synaptic transmission and the maintenance of membrane potential always seem to iron out differences and return the system to a constant resting state.

There are thus good and widespread mechanisms for short-term modification of nervous transmission dependent in a proportional manner on the recent history of impulse activity, over a period of seconds, and lasting for up to half an hour or so. So widespread are these events among neurones that a learning mechanism would certainly have to take account of them, if it did not use one or a combination as an immediate store of the history of recent activity.

SIMPLE SYSTEMS FOR THE STUDY OF SYNAPTIC CONNECTIVITY AND RHYTHMICAL BEHAVIOUR

Anything that is discovered about the mechanisms of synaptic transmission is potentially applicable to the phenomenon of memory, specially those effects that outlast the immediate consequences of stimulation and influence the subsequent behaviour. Apart from the neuromuscular junction and certain very large synapses in the nervous system of invertebrates (Katz and Miledi, 1970) from which most of our detailed knowledge of the physiology of synapses has stemmed there are a host of more complex situations where the techniques of intracellular or extracellular unit recording and controlled electrical stimulation of pre-synaptic pathways make an analysis of interneuronal signalling possible. The simpler pathways through the mammalian spinal cord (Thompson and Spencer, 1966; Wickelgren, 1967; Spencer and April, 1970), the relatively small collections of nerve cells of the ganglia of invertebrate nervous systems (Kandel and Tauc, 1965), activity of the mammalian cerebral cortex (Morrell, Engel, and Bouris, 1967) and many other preparations can be managed in acute electrophysiological experiments and the response of selected nerve cells correlated with the stimulation of various pre-synaptic pathways.

Sometimes the electrophysiological analysis of these preparations is done by setting the sequences of stimulation of various pre-synaptic pathways to mimic the sequence of presentation of a conditioned and unconditioned stimulus in a classical conditioned reflex experiment in a whole animal. The experiment is often then described as an attempt to find a simple system for the study of learning and great attention given to the modification of effectiveness of one pre-synaptic stimulus by pairing with another.

In some invertebrate ganglia changes occur that do greatly resemble learning of the whole animal (Luco and Aranda, 1964). An isolated metathoracic ganglion of a locust and the leg it controls can be set up in a learning experiment and the leg trained to maintain a fixed posture by punishing deviations from the chosen position by electric shocks. Horridge (1962) in this experiment used another locust leg as a control, yoked in series with the shock source attached to the learning leg. This second leg could also move in response to nervous commands from its own ganglion but the shock would be delivered apparently at random, and not contingent upon any constant position of the leg as would be the case for the learning preparation. Both legs had very similar experiences but learning emerged from the leg in which shock did have a constant relationship to leg positions. Hoyle (1965) has shown that motor axons in the absence of the leg can also learn in the same way to hold a preferred frequency of discharge. This looked as though it would be a most useful preparation but the idea received a set-back when Eisenstein and Cohen (1965) found that a preparation from which the nerve ganglia had been removed could also learn just about as well as an innervated one. Only by using Horridge's yoked control technique could it be seen that the contingency-specific pattern of response was absent in the deganglionated leg. Its behaviour changed when shocked and was long-lasting but was due to some other modification in the peripheral nervous system or muscles, not to learning in the ganglion, which by itself accounts for only part, although the critical part, of the modification of behaviour. Indeed from the records it appears that the function of the nervous system in the ganglion may be to prevent the occurrence of response modification in peripheral structures unless time relations between stimulus and response are appropriate. Similar interrelations between the central nervous system and peripheral organs occur in the learning of siphon withdrawal in mollusc Aplysia (Lukowiak and Jacklett, 1972).

Attempts to modify the conductivity through networks of neurones in the mammalian cortex which have been isolated from the rest of the brain by anatomical disconnection, leaving the blood supply intact, have very often been successful. The complexity of the interneuronal pathways means that electrical stimuli applied to either of two separate regions of the isolated cortex, stimulating separate bundles of nerve fibres, can be made to make a single common neurone fire, as registered by its unitary action potential. Most pathways show a depression of conductance (the neurone gives a progressively weaker response with repeated stimuli). If conditioning stimuli are applied through one pathway for several minutes the response to stimuli through the other pathway is often increased, sometimes for long periods of at least thirty minutes and perhaps indefinitely. Opposite changes are also seen (Bliss, Burns, and Uttley, 1968). In the hippocampal cortex, stimulation of one pathway can lead to prolonged increases in the efficacy of this one alone (Bliss and Lømo, 1970).

No one knows the functions that these isolated networks of cortical neurones normally perform or whether they ever come together functionally during life. Neither is the anatomical connectivity, particularly in the neocortex, clear, nor are the physiological routes of excitation and inhibition. These facts, which are well known to the experimenters, pre-

clude any direct extrapolation of these results to the phenomenon of whole animal learning but they do not detract from
the interest of such demonstrations of the nature and extent
of the potential modifiability of neuronal networks, as they
naturally occur. In other cortical areas in the intact animal
repeated pairing of visual and auditory stimuli both of which
initially influenced the firing of one cortical neurone would
eventually modify the response of the neurone to one of the
stimuli alone, the effect lasting about thirty minutes (Morrell,
Engel, and Bouris, 1967).

Another use of both vertebrate and invertebrate preparations is to study the apparently spontaneous rhythmic activity
of nerve cells which is also a prominent property of higher
nervous systems, and as explained in Chapter 1, could
also provide a mechanism for permanent change of neuronal
networks. Isolated cells in invertebrate ganglia can keep up
rhythmic activity in the absence of all synaptic input and
the regulation may be under quite direct genetic control since
the appropriate anti-metabolites can interfere with rhythm-
icity (Strumwasser, 1964). Artificial stimuli, or natural ones
applied to the living animal, such as a shift in its light–dark
cycle, can reset the rhythmic behaviour of neurones which
will continue to respond to the same period after many days
in culture outside the animal (Lickey, 1969).

In neurones of the rat cerebral cortex it is possible when the
conditions of anaesthesia are right to produce long-lasting
changes in the firing pattern of single neurones by passing
quite a weak direct current in the appropriate direction
through the cortex for a few minutes (Bindman, Lippold, and
Redfearn, 1962). These changes last for hours and are also
sensitive to anti-metabolites acting on mechanisms of protein
synthesis (Gartside, 1968b).

The effects can be shown to depend upon some memory of
the induced firing pattern of the cell, not upon the polarizing
current (Bindman and Boisacq-Scheppens, 1966), and once
developed will survive interruption of firing by cooling and
rewarming or other transient disruption of function of the
cortex (Gartside, 1968a). A difference between this phenomenon and memory is mainly the long time required for its
induction, more than five minutes and about 2000 stimuli.

The final analysis of this could, however, be as complicated as that for behavioural memory since many thousands of cortical circuits acting in series or in parallel could be involved in the regulation of the rhythmic firing of any one cortical neurone. Without anaesthesia the cells do not seem to have modifiable behaviour (Boisacq-Scheppens, 1968). Anaesthetic dependent changes in firing pattern of spinal cord neurones, that resemble changes in the cortex have also been described (Melzack, Konrad, and Dubrovsky, 1969).

Each of these examples of physiological flexibility must have its proper biological meaning. There must be a lot of learning in the lower reaches of the nervous system as well as in the parts of the brain more obviously concerned with the behaviour of the whole animal. Even the simplest reflex actions may have some mechanism for monitoring their effectiveness and updating the parameters of action according to their success. Horridge (1967) has described such a situation in the control of optokinetic reflexes of the crab eye. The analysis of these processes loses clarity when they are forced to take on a most unsuitable role as a model for the adaptive behaviour of the whole animal.

The use of simple systems

The problem in neurophysiology then is not to find the modifiable synapse or neurone. There are already too many of them, particularly if one takes into account experiments on habituation to repeated stimuli (Horn, 1970). Almost any neurophysiological preparation, even the neuromuscular junction itself can be set up to demonstrate changes in responsiveness dependent upon the history of use. However, in neurophysiology almost all such preparations that do change in an obvious manner contain an enormous number of cells, synapses, and potential circuits for impulse activity and often require some extra manipulation, anaesthesia, surgical isolation, or the like.

Our knowledge of the physiology of excitable membranes and of synaptic transmission has in fact depended upon the intensive study of a few selected preparations that do not show much in the way of use-dependent changes, the giant axon of the squid (Hodgkin, 1964), the vertebrate neuromuscular junction (Katz, 1969), and the simplest reflex synaptic connections of the cat spinal cord (Eccles, 1969). Once we get away from these preparations, to something with only a few more cells and synapses, rigorous experiments of the kind that have generated the basic neurophysiological knowledge are no longer possible. Effects can be seen and measured, described and reproduced, but the final mechanistic explanation, compatible with the very high level of scientific excellence set by the pioneers of fundamental neurophysiology, is rarely attainable. Indeed the notion of a simple system almost anywhere in the nervous system is not realistic. Synaptic connections are too small and packed together so densely ($10^{12}/cm^{-3}$ in the cerebral cortex) that it takes only a fragment of nervous tissue to perform the most complicated control functions. There are insects so small that they could crawl up the inside of a squid giant axon, and yet they have a nervous system that can cope with sensation, locomotion, orientation, feeding, mating, and probably a lot of learning (Vowles, 1965). A goldfish optic lobe, in those commonly used in the laboratory for learning experiments, is about the size of a pinhead, although not as thick through. It is a good bet that visual memories of the most complicated type can be stored here, just as in the octopus optic lobe (Mark, Peer, and Steiner, 1973). When one considers the complexity and subtlety of fish visuomotor behaviour one would have no right to connect up electrodes to, say, the optic nerves as input and the tecto-bulbar tract as output and imply one was dealing with a simple system for anything.

Nevertheless experiments of the kind so briefly described in this chapter, but well reviewed elsewhere (Kandel and Spencer, 1968; Cragg, 1972), are important to do now because they generate ideas about the modifiability of neuronal function, ideas which were deliberately excluded from the classical experiments of cellular neurophysiology. Some of these findings may be relevant to memory but in no case as yet has the complete analysis of the synaptic mechanism been possible.

THEORETICAL MEMORY CIRCUITS

A quite separate avenue of memory research, which is rapidly becoming important for physiology, is the theoretical.

A crucial paper in 1967 by Brindley collected together and described the logical structure of various theoretical networks of neurone-like elements that would show the properties of Pavlovian conditioned reflexes, with the possibility of extinction. An extension of this work (Gardner-Medwin, 1969) showed that if bursts of impulses rather than single spikes were the normal form of signalling between such elements, the constraints for the kind of network capable of learning from experience became different, and different again if spontaneous activity was permitted. A network can be constructed with only one synapse, the function of which changes with use, and able to account for learning and extinction. With a cumulative effect of learning experiences on the one modifiable element consolidation could occur (Brindley, 1969). It emphasizes the possibility that in the real brain modifiable elements may be rare to begin with and the elements that change during a particular learning experience rarer still. Of course natural nervous networks with their tremendous interconnectivity and the parallel organization of thousands of channels bear no immediate resemblance to models that may be easily manipulated by logical analysis, but useful principles can be discovered in this way (McCulloch and Pitts, 1943; Griffith, 1966; Longuet-Higgins, Willshaw, and Buneman, 1970).

The theoretical analysis of real networks is also more fruitful nowadays that detailed anatomy and the disposition of excitatory and inhibitory synapses is now more or less known for some brain regions. It is therefore possible to make more progress than Cajal who interpreted all connections as excitatory, and the analysis is being attempted by people with a better mathematical knowledge than he. There are several theories for the cerebellum (Albus, 1971; Marr, 1969) and coherent theories for neocortex and archicortex which includes the hippocampus (Marr, 1970, 1971). They include specific ideas as to which should be the modifiable elements in order that learning should occur, given current knowledge of connectivity and synapse function. These predictions are exact enough for experimental test, which brings brain science close in line with the physical sciences, where the two modes of theoretical prediction and practical test are carried out by

separate individual or research groups. Such work, theoretical
and practical, can specify the class of cell or synapse that should
change its behaviour in order to modify input–output relations of a network but cannot discover the biochemical mechanism for change, or the nature of the regulatory mechanisms
that guard some elements against change while maintaining
the permanence of change in others.

AND WHAT NOW?

There are thus many ways in which the results of research
on neurobiology can be brought to bear on the question of
the nature of memory. However it would be less than honest
to end the exposition of this phase of the argument with the
idea that in the author's opinion all these modes of attack are
equally useful. On the contrary, in spite of much fine work
and in spite of the importance of experiments noted in this
chapter for the historical development of physiological memory research, many lines now pursued seem unlikely to home
in on a really powerful explanation of the mechanisms of
adaptive behaviour.

It is now more than ten years since Horridge (1962) described the apparent learning ability of the locust ganglion,
still one of the best experiments of its kind, in the hope that
analysis of this preparation would reveal the physiological
mechanism of its adaptable behaviour. In 1972 Farel and
Buerger described the same procedure carried out successfully
(and not for the first time (Horn and Horn, 1969)) in the frog
spinal cord and they end their paper this way, 'Because of
its relative anatomical simplicity this preparation may be very
useful in analysing the anatomical, physiological, and biochemical mechanisms of learning.' True enough perhaps, but
if nothing has happened in the last ten years it is because we
still have no idea of what kind of neuronal change to expect.
Some new physiological principles must be brought into thinking about the cellular nature of learning so that this kind of
experiment can be given a new framework for interpretation
and more penetrating experiments can be designed.

6 A Theory of Modifiable Brain Cell Networks

IF a lack of independently observable mechanisms for permanent modifiability in the mechanism of impulse communication between cells leads us away from this process as the basis of long-term changes in brain function, the undeniable importance of the fine details of functional interneuronal connections in all aspects of brain function studied leads us back again to the pattern of synaptic connectivity as the main mechanism for orderly function of the brain. A clue as to the modifiability of the brain is therefore likely to be found within the laws which describe the development of detailed interneuronal connections, those patterns that are read out so faithfully year after year by the biophysical mechanism of synaptic transmission.

NERVE REGENERATION EXPERIMENTS AND THE CONCEPT OF GRADIENTS

The early observations of Weiss and Sperry, amplified and refined by later workers show that the return of brain function after regeneration of severed axonal sprouts can only be due to the reformation of terminal synaptic relations with an accuracy approaching or equalling that of initial morphogenetic development. It is also clear that much of the formation of specific synaptic connections does not require use or practice, but follows developmental signals that serve to match up populations of neurones before nervous connections between them are completed, as between motoneurones and muscles, or between retinal ganglion cells and the optic lobe of the brain. During development both of these sets of neurones undergo a parallel differentiation that not only sets the cell types and their articulation into the surrounding nervous network but also serves to distinguish them from their neighbours.

The physical basis of such specificity is not known but in the explanation of all these experimental results use has been made of the idea of an embryological marker which is carried by adult cells and contains information not just as to the kind of cell but as to its place in a network of similar cells. The idea is common in embryology where the placement of a cell may condition the developmental line it generates and so the shape and structure of the tissue or the organism (Wolpert, 1969). Such developmental space-coding appears to arrive in embryogenesis early on by the operation of mechanisms that rely upon a diffusion gradient set up across a population of a relatively small number of cells packed in an area of less than a square millimetre (Crick, 1970). The information somehow becomes set into the early cells at a critical period and then expands with cell division to regulate the morphogenesis of much larger areas.

Cell recognition that may be identified in other systems, for example by specific reaggregation of dispersed cultured cells, or antigen recognition by lymphocytes, depends somehow upon the mucopolysaccharide cell coat on the outside of the membrane which has been postulated to have a specific molecular conformation that can recognize corresponding cells or molecules (Lilien, 1969). Certainly there is an abundance of protein polysaccharide in the brain on neuronal surfaces, concentrated even in the gap between pre- and post-synaptic cell membranes at the point where interneuronal recognition must be translated into a structural form. In the present state of knowledge, however, it is better not to argue too far by analogy until some definite information comes from neuroembryology as to what kind of molecules subserve neuronal specificity. Such molecules should include protein because the delicacy of the distinctions made by growing synapses in the formation of functional interneuronal connections seems to demand a molecular mechanism of great flexibility and information capacity. Perhaps each cell has a specific marker protein, perhaps many in varying proportions, perhaps distributed unevenly about the cell. There is no point in being precise about matters that are now theoretical constructs that only serve to make sense of cellular function and cannot yet be put into a form in which experimental test of the various combinations becomes possible.

The question then arises as to whether all this is done in one developmental episode in embryonic foetal and neonatal life and then the gene pool is covered for ever, or whether the maintenance of such a highly ordered piece of matter as the brain requires continual metabolic effort. The latter is almost certainly true because the rate of manufacture of structural protein in the mammalian brain, as measured by incorporation and turnover of radioactivity labelled amino acids into protein, is as high as that in the liver and higher than any other tissue in the adult body. Yet the brain does not grow in size, neurones do not divide and it has no metabolic protein output such as the plasma proteins from the liver. Therefore the protein synthesis must be balanced by a correspondingly high rate of protein breakdown (Lajtha, 1970).

The reason for such rapid turnover of structural molecules in an organ that remains macroscopically the same size and microscopically apparently unchanging for year after year of adult life is not known. Since there is no other apparent reason, it seems probable that there is constant manufacture, exchange, and recognition of, and response of neurones to, specific protein-containing marker molecules that maintain or modify, within tight limits set by the developmental mechanisms, the detailed pattern of functional intercellular synaptic connections. It is quite possible that none of this results in overt morphological change, recognizable even by the electron microscope.

It is difficult for a neurophysiologist, who has the most intimate knowledge of neurone function, to accept that the cells, which are visible to him as the highly predictable generators of patterns of transmembrane or extracellular electric current flows, also contain such an incredibly detailed record of their embryological origin and present place in a vast three-dimensional lattice of interconnected cells. Perhaps if the moment-to-moment behaviour of the brain was quite independent of the developmental mechanisms that set up these patterns in the first place this would not matter but a series of experiments on the neurophysiology of developing sensory pathways show that the use of a set of neurones does influence the maintenance of connections established by developmental processes.

NEURONAL USE THAT DOES PRODUCE PERMANENT CHANGES *Frogs*

The most recently discovered, but the best described, of these situations is the growth of binocular connections from the eye to the brain in frogs and toads. These animals have a retina rather like that of the mammals in neuronal organization and it projects by a completely crossed optic nerve to the optic lobe of the mid-brain on the opposite side. The growth of connections between retinal ganglion cells and the optic tectum is regulated by the same developmental processes that have been described in Chapter 3. Ganglion cells and optic lobe neurones must undergo a parallel differentiation quite early on in the embryological development and the connections between the two groups of ordered neurones follows this differentiation. The result of this process is a point-to-point connection of retina to optic lobe (Gaze, 1958).

These animals also have a central projection of the retina on to the optic lobe of the same side by a pathway that passes through the contralateral optic lobe and via an interneuronal relay that crosses from one tectum to another over the post-optic commissures to generate another projection on the ipsilateral optic lobe. Careful mapping of these two projections shows the ipsilateral and contralateral projection to be perfectly in register on each side when the optic axes of the two eyes are in normal position. Therefore every object in space in front of the animal has a double representation on each optic lobe of the mid-brain, reaching there through both eyes. The exact corresponding spot of the double representation on the brain is different for all visual loci except for the strip of visual space directly in front of the animals. For this area each spot in space projects to symmetrical points on the optic lobes, each side receiving information from each eye (Gaze and Jacobson, 1962).

The development of the interneuronal ipsilateral projection of the visual field shows features relevant to memory. In order for the two projections of the visual field to be in register on each side there must be an interneuronal commissure, a transverse nerve-fibre pathway connecting the two tecta so that the disposition of images is reversed as the information goes from one lobe to another. This must be so because although the geometry of the primary projection, medial field to anterior tectum, lateral field to posterior tectum, is the same on each side, an image from an object in front of the animal is not symmetrically represented in each eye. The object to the left of the animal falls on the medial retina on the *left* eye and the lateral retina of the right eye. Following the common projection pattern for each eye it can be seen that the representation of the common object will be the opposite way round on each tectum (Fig. 8a) (Keating and Gaze, 1970).

If one eye is removed during development of these animals contralateral projection from the remaining eye is normal, but the ipsilateral projection is distorted. Instead of the discrete projection usually found, many spots in the visual field can excite an evoked potential at many tectal positions. The projection is therefore diffuse, each place in the visual field being multiply represented on the optic lobe, although the overall order of projection is still recognizable. This must mean that the neurones that normally make up the intertectal commissure no longer project to such discrete places on the opposite optic lobe but branch more extensively to generate evoked potentials at a large number of terminal loci. If one eye is inverted or rotated in the skull at a time after the embryological gradients have become established (see Chapter 3) a further modification of the ipsilateral projection on each side is seen. It develops but the ipsilateral projection on each side is once again in register with the contralateral projection. This occurs in spite of the contralateral projection showing the rotation expected from translocation of the eye at this early stage of development. It can only mean that the intertectal projection was modified at some stage in the animal's life so that it matched the distorted projection from the operated eye. Thus if one eye is inverted the two contralateral projections would not be crossed images of each other but mirror images with the same point in visual space represented at symmetrical points on the optic lobe. When the intertectal crossing fails to develop, each point on one tectum connects to the directly opposite point of the other tectum. On each

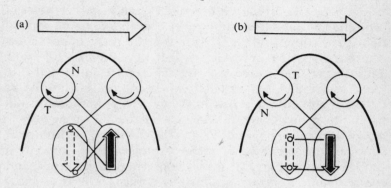

FIG. 8. Binocular projection of the visual field on to the optic lobe of a frog. (*a*) Normal projection to the right tectum, directly from the left eye and indirectly via the left tectum and the crossed inter-tectal pathway from the right eye. (*b*) The effect of inverting the left eye in early development. The projection via this eye to the right tectum is inverted. When the indirect pathway from the right eye develops, it is also inverted to match, even though the direct projection from this eye to the left tectum is in the normal orientation. (After Gaze, Keating, Szekeley, and Beazley, 1970.)

side therefore the two projections, one from each eye, on to the optic lobe are once again in register (Gaze, Keating, Szekely, and Beazley, 1970) (Fig. 8b).

The complete experimental conditions for producing this phenomenon appear not to be completely understood because at least one attempt to repeat the observations is reported to have failed (Jacobson, 1971).

The important matter that emerges from the cases where inverted projections do develop is that in attempting to explain this it is no use to follow the rules laid down earlier which require parallel differentiation of two sets of neurones. Now it is the neurones from the normal tectum that modify their terminations in the opposite abnormal tectum to ensure congruous excitation in that abnormal projection (Keating, 1968). The easiest hypothesis to explain it all is that the neurones that form the ipsilateral relayed projection were originally diffuse in their projection to the relevant neurones of the optic lobe on the other side. Each of these cells would therefore receive two visual inputs, one from the direct contralateral projection from the opposite eye and another series of projections from a large number of branches of neurones participating in the ipsilateral projection from the opposite tectum but connected synaptically to the eye on the same side. This appears to be the primitive state of the ipsilateral projection since this is what is left when one eye is removed or indeed if animals are raised in the dark so vision cannot contribute to neurogenesis (Feldman, Gaze, and Keating, 1971). An object in the visual field will therefore excite tectal neurones through both of these pathways, one contralateral and laid down by genetic or developmental mechanisms, and one ipsilateral following an initially diffuse pathway to many cells and the opposite tectum. The adult pattern is no longer diffuse, therefore many of the early projections must be lost. Those remaining will be the ones that lead to the cell on the contralateral tectum that receives excitation from the same point in visual space. Therefore, of the multiple connections of this interneurone, only those synapses are retained that are used in synergy with the direct projection from the contralateral eye. All other synaptic terminations of this neurone and those that would not be active in synergy with the converging synapses from the direct contralateral projection are lost. Yet these other diverging projections are active at a time when the contralateral projections are silent without apparently influencing their maintenance. Ipsilateral and contralateral synapses on to tectal neurones are apparently not therefore equal in value in resisting the influence of converging projections. Contralateral projections are retained no matter what the concurrent pattern of activity in converging interneuronal projections. But the intertectal connections are only retained if they are active at the same time as the primary projection from the opposite eye. If, as seems highly likely these two sets of synapses terminate on one neurone they must interchange information as to their origin, whether from the eye or the opposite tectum, and on this information depends the retention or loss of synaptic terminations. Ipsilateral terminations are vulnerable but can persist if they transmit every time the contralateral synapses do, if not they are lost (Fig. 9).

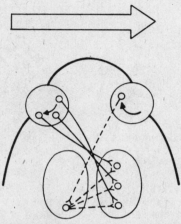

FIG. 9. Possible mechanism of selection of the correct intertectal synaptic connections. Each locus on the left tectum has potential connections with many positions on the opposite tectum. Those connections from the cell shown to the opposite anterior tectum will be fired off in conjunction with the direct projection from the opposite eye. This means they will be retained. Other potential connections are lost because they do not fire in conjunction with the direct connections, which can suppress convergent synapses through a more powerful chemotrophic action.

Simple visual responses of tadpoles

A similar phenomenon occurs in the development of simple reflex responses of tadpoles to slow movements of the visual field. Normally the animals respond by turning gently so as to fix the moving world on the eye. Each eye contributes to turning responses of the whole body when the visual movement is from back to front of the animal (that is, from the temporal to nasal visual fields) but scarcely at all for movements in the opposite direction. If one eye is removed, or simply rotated 90° in the head so that discordant impulse patterns are produced, the visual reaction of the untouched eye improves so that it becomes responsible for turning movements in both directions (Fig. 10). The pattern of use of the visual input from the rotated eye has therefore influenced the functional neuronal connections made by the untouched normal eye (Mark and Feldman, 1972). The mechanism of this change could be similar to that for development of binocular connections in the tectum but must be elsewhere in the

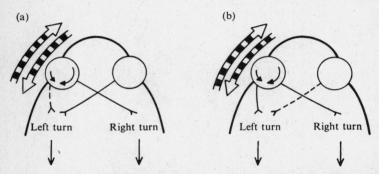

FIG. 10. Mechanism of direction sensitivity in optokinetic reflexes. (*a*) Normally each eye is mainly sensitive to temporal-to-nasal movement, which produces movement of the eyes and head to the right. Movement the other way evokes very weak responses. (*b*) After removal or rotation of one eye early in development the normal eye becomes powerful at driving in both directions. Therefore previously ineffective connections have become more effective in the absence of competitive impulses from the opposite eye. (After Mark and Feldman, 1972.)

brain because such simple visual responses do not require the optic lobes at all. Probably both eyes have potential connections to movement-producing systems for left and right turning. Normally, for example, nerve cells from the right eye develop the strongest connections on neurones which control movement of the body to the left. These nerve terminals may compete with the fewer or less effective nerve cells from the opposite eye for control of common post-synaptic movement producing neurones. The terminals that are normally disadvantaged in development may assume complete control if function of the normally dominant ones is disorganized (Fig. 10).

Binocular vision in cats

Similar events go to make up the binocular projection from the two eyes of mammals and cells of the visual cortex. The pathway in this case is from the retinal ganglion cells of the eye through the optic nerve to the lateral geniculate nucleus in the thalamus. This nucleus is a laminated structure with terminals from the two eyes ending on geniculate cells in different layers. These cells send axons to the back of the cerebral cortex, the occipital lobe where single axons from the pathway from the two eyes converge on the same post-synaptic neurone.

The geometry of these projections has a most interesting detailed organization. The site of termination of the retinal ganglion cell axons in the thalamus depends on their position to the left or right of a line drawn through the centre of the eye from dorsal to ventral. The axons from these ganglion cells on the medial side of this division cross to the opposite side of the brain to end in the contralateral lateral geniculate nucleus, those to the outside of the division of the retina remain on the same side. Now if the eyes are side by side at the front of the head, then an image thrown on to both retinae by an object in front of the animal will be similarly inverted by the simple optics of the eye in both the up and down and left and right directions. In the up and down direction the transformation is the same for both eyes but in the left–right transformation the same part of the object will appear on the medial side of one eye and the lateral side of the other.

The system of separate crossing pathways for the medial hemiretina ganglion cell axons restores the congruency of images, so that projections from the right and left visual yields in front of the animal are found together in the lateral geniculate of each side. But the pathways through this nucleus remain neurologically separated by the layered structure of this collection of neurones. At the visual cortex axons from the separate layers of geniculate neurones come together on to the same cortical cell so that objects in space, which form images in both eyes, generate impulses which end up exciting precisely the same cerebral cortical neurones (Fig 11) (Hubel and Wiesel, 1962).

This convergence of corresponding points on the retina to

single cortical neurones is important in the mechanism of distance judgement and three-dimensional vision for which two frontally placed eyes are so important. So important is the precise correspondence of the neurological wiring with the optical projections in the two eyes from single points in space that the

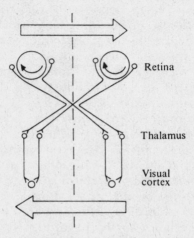

Fig. 11. The arrangement of the neuronal pathway from the retina to the visual cortex of mammals. Images from both sides of the mid-line of the visual field fall on both eyes. Points receiving corresponding images in each eye give rise to pathways that converge on common neurones in the visual cortex.

development of these connections apparently depends partly on the use of this system in early life as well as on genetic developmental instructions for ordering neuronal connections. This appears to be so because, if the vision in one eye is occluded during a critical early period of a kitten's life, the convergence of excitation from two eyes on to common cortical neurones is permanently lost (Wiesel and Hubel, 1963). There are still many cortical cells connected to the visual system but they are divided into two population groups, one connected to each eye, instead of the majority being connected to two, as is usual. Visual occlusion is not necessary to produce this developmental abnormality. The retinal images in the two eyes have only to be made not to correspond, which can be done by daily alternate occlusion of the eyes (Wiesel and

Hubel, 1965a) or by inducing án artificial squint by surgically cutting one of the muscles that move the eye (Hubel and Wiesel, 1965). Clinical experience has long recognized the dependence of vision of a cross-eye on the early correction of the squint (Phillip, 1965). A turning eye not treated will eventually lose vision completely. The explanation appears to lie partly in a failure of the cortical connections of such an eye to be maintained (Wiesel and Hubel, 1965b; Dews and Wiesel, 1970). How could such a fine selection of the best converging synaptic connections of cortical visual neurones be achieved?

Obviously the gross, and much of the fine patterning of the neuronal connections is under genetic control because it occurs early in development before vision and is present in good order at birth and in animals that have never been outside the uterus. However, the initial connections of geniculate-to-cortical neurones are more widespread. Each cortical neurone will receive a large number of connections from geniculate cells representing an area in visual space seen in common by each eye. Now assume that if two terminals on such a cell are activated synchronously they will be retained together, if they are active at odd times one or the other, perhaps the strongest, will not be retained. The result will be the retention of pairs of synaptic terminations from opposite eyes arising from retinal ganglion cells that reflect precisely the same visual events, that is from parts of the retina lined up with the same spot in visual space. It is the same postulated mechanism for development of the ipsilateral visual projection in the toad, and again we have no idea of how it could be brought about in terms of nerve cells.

Receptive fields of neurones of the cat visual cortex

The cells that show binocular correspondence are also very finely space-coded for the precise visual stimulus that serves to excite them. They respond best to bars or edges of contrasting illumination moved in a particular direction at a restricted location of the visual field. This behaviour results from the patterning of neuronal connections from the retina to the cortex so that a set of retinal photoreceptor cells arranged in a band across a small region of the retina comes to have unique control of the cortical neurones.

Animals that are raised so that all the contours of the visual world are in one direction, a world of only horizontal and vertical stripes, develop a predominance of cortical cells that respond to the predominant environmental contours. The animals' behavioural responses show the same changes. They are blind to contours they have never seen (Blakemore and Cooper, 1970; Hirsch and Spinnelli, 1971; Hirsch, 1972; Spinelli, Hirsch, Phelps, and Metzler, 1972).

Such a finding can be explained in the same way. Contour specificity in cortical cells comes about by a competition for common post-synaptic neurones by many nerve terminals from the next cells back in the chain. In the absence of strong environmental pressures the embryologically determined pattern is established. Strong or continued activity of a minority of connections could disrupt the unused convergent connections, even though developmentally they may be the preferred ones (Hubel and Wiesel, 1963, but see Barlow and Pettigrew, 1971).

Amphibian limbs

The principle of supplying, by growth, an overabundance of nerve cells or synaptic connections and fixing the final patterns by discarding many of them seems to show up often in the development of the nervous system, specially in the finer details of connection formation. Similar things happen in neuromuscular connections in the development of amphibia where there is good and carefully collected evidence that many extra nerve cells differentiate in the spinal cord as the limbs begin to be formed and that many of these send axons out to the muscles. As the stage of limb movement arrives many of these cells die so that the final number of motoneurones is much smaller than the number of cells genetically capable of this function (Hughes, 1968; Prestige, 1970). In this case there is no doubt that unsuccessful motoneurones actually die and are lost from the nervous system. Animals deprived of the pituitary at this stage of development are left with a larger than usual number of motor nerve fibres suggesting that death depends on some hormonal influence.

Gaining successful peripheral connections with a muscle confers resistance to the lethal action of a hormone, perhaps from the thyroid (Race, 1961).

PRINCIPLES OF DETAILED CONNECTION FORMATION

These few examples of brain development have been chosen and explained in detail because they show a common pattern in the formation of cell networks in which precision of connection is critical for proper function. Innate developmental mechanisms do most of the work in getting the correct cell types connected with each other. The number of connections is larger than will be required and the distribution more diffuse than in the final product. In the examples from the visual system, the final selection procedure involves simultaneous use of converging projections, or synapses and those used in isolation disappear. With motoneurones it is unclear whether function is required for the selection, but in common with the visual examples it is clear that the final pattern depends on growing too many cells and dispensing with those that are not useful.

The plasticity of synaptic connection related to use in these cases is not an enhancement of efficacy but a competitive suppression of transmission from other converging connections. The final pattern emerges not because the best-fitted connections improve but because the inappropriate are eliminated.

These examples of modified neuronal connection come from developmental episodes which terminate in a permanent nervous network much better than the product of first growth. Could such a process, under some circumstance, be prolonged into adult life and continue to modify brain connections into a more appropriate form for current experience?

The development of binocular vision in mammals, cats, and man is a specially clear example as there is a critical period for the loss of connections which sets the pattern for life (Hubel and Wiesel, 1970). If this were to be a model for memory in adult animals the critical period would have to be lifelong. Also we must take account of the fact that no anatomical search for brain changes in memory has discovered anything of importance. Any changes related to learning are likely to be very slight at the light-microscopic, or even at the electronmicroscopic level because, with all the work that has so far gone into neurohistology by itself and in relation to changes in behaviour, if something as obvious as cell or terminal degeneration was required one feels that some evidence should have shown up by now. It has not, so if this kind of modifiability is used in lifelong learning, it seems to occur through molecular changes that are not yet visible microscopically.

One test for admission of this theory is therefore as follows: can growth controlling processes, that operate in the selection of interneuronal synaptic connections control synaptic transmissions without any discernible morphological correlation? This is exactly what does happen in the selection of the correct motoneurone terminals in re-innervation of multiply-innervated eye muscles in fish. The continuation of Weiss' and Sperry's work on recovery of co-ordination after random regeneration of cut nerve fibres, outlined in Chapter 3 has shown clearly that the mechanisms controlling connection formation are much less selective than the mechanisms regulating transmission from the formed synapses. An eye muscle will accept terminals which appear normal by electron microscopy from an antagonist nerve and contract in response to impulses in the nerve. Only when the correctly marked nerve grows back into the muscle these synapses lose their efficacy and yet show no discernible signs of degeneration (Marotte and Mark, 1970) (Fig. 12). Neither do the motoneurones change appreciably in their reflex behaviour, for impulses may be recorded from the motor axons as they enter the muscle even when no contraction occurs (Mark and Marotte, 1972).

This observation provides the precedent that growth-controlling recognition mechanisms, of the kind thought to underly the normal development of interneuronal connections, may also control the transmission at formed synaptic connections, by competitive means which do not cause immediate degeneration and loss of suppressed synapses (Mark, Marotte, and Mart 1972). The biophysical reason for suppressed transmission is not yet known. Suppression of synaptic transmission in a muscle does not seem to depend on relative use of synapses. Both correct and incorrect nerves should be equally active.

Another set of experiments on neuromuscular innervation in axolotl limbs shows the same process of repression of innervation to be reversible and also begins to suggest that use of

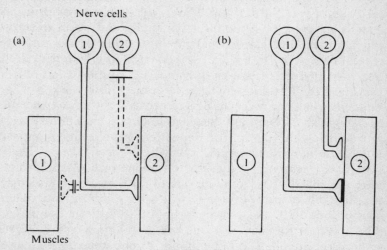

FIG. 12. Experiments on the selection of correct connections between nerves and muscles of fish eyes. (*a*) Nerve 1, originally controlling muscle 1, is transplanted into muscle 2 whose own nerve is cut near the nerve cell bodies. Nerve 1 gains functional synaptic contact and causes muscle 2 to contract. (*b*) Nerve 2 grows back from the cell body and reforms synaptic connections with muscle 2. When this happens the synaptic connections from nerve 1 onto muscle 2 stop transmitting. The terminals of nerve 1 still appear normal by electronmicroscopy. (After Marotte and Mark, 1970.)

synapses may be as important as their presence in maintaining effective connectivity.

If the nerves supplying a limb are cut and reimplanted into the wrong part of the root of the limb, they grow widely during regeneration but eventually end up innervating the correct muscles. This can be seen by observing the muscular contraction after stimulating various nerves, as has been done by Grimm (1971), or by making a detailed map of the location of effective neuromuscular synapses by recording their electrical signs of junctional transmission with an intracellular microelectrode, as has been done by Cass and Mark (1972).

The restoration of the correct pattern of neuromuscular connections must be an expression of a process of selective affinity
between nerve and muscle cells similar to that between nerve
cells in the brain. By cutting only one of the three main nerves
that supply a leg, the terminals of the remaining nerves can
be encouraged to grow into the freshly denervated muscle
(Stirling, 1973; Sutton and Mark, 1973). New synaptic terminals are formed in the foreign muscles and begin to transmit, a process that takes about three weeks (Fig. 13). Eventually
the cut nerve grows back, and as it does the foreign innervation
becomes ineffective, just as in competitive innervation of fish
eye muscles. The interesting extension of this work is what
happens when the regrown nerve is cut a second time and the
mapping experiments are done again. Before and immediately
after cutting the nerve, the dependent muscle fibres appear
to have no functional connections with adjacent nerves. However if the mapping experiment is done two to three days
after cutting the nerve the muscle fibres that were previously
supplied by it are found already to have strong functional
connections with the nerve that supplies adjacent muscles.
The first time the nerve was cut and innervation was observed
to spread into denervated muscle it took three weeks and
occurred mainly, it appears, by growth of new nerve sprouts.
If the spread of innervation takes only three days the second
time, this surely means that the new foreign connections did
not disappear upon competitive innervation but were simply
functionally repressed. Removal of the correct innervation
allows them to become functional once more.

If the nerve terminals in these limbs are examined by the
electron miscroscope at intervals after cutting their axon it is
found that three days is barely time for the process of structural
degeneration to have begun (Mart and Mark, 1972). One
wonders then whether the effect of nerve section that leads to
a reawakening of dormant synapses from other convergent
nerves might be the absence of impulse activity in the
severed axon. Indeed, Aguilar, Bisby, and Diamond (1972)
working with another species of salamander have reported
that spread of innervation, both sensory and motor, will occur
when impulse activity in the nerve trunk is blocked by a local
anaesthetic or when intracellular transport of material in the

axon is blocked, without interfering with impulse activity. Thus both the electrical activity of a terminal and metabolic products delivered to it from the cell body may be important in maintaining its influence on the muscle and presumably its repressive influence on converging mismatched connections.

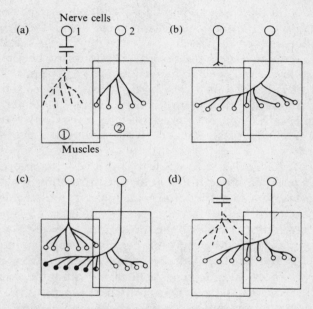

FIG. 13. Further experiments on formation of functional connections between nerves and muscles in salamander limbs. (*a*) Muscle 1 is denervated. (*b*) Nerves from muscle 2 grow into muscle 1 and form functional synaptic connections. This takes several weeks. (*c*) When the correct nerves grow back to muscle 1 the foreign innervation stops working but the connections remain in the muscle as repressed synapses. (*d*) If nerve 1 is cut again these connections are derepressed and begin to transmit again. This takes two or three days. (After Cass, Sutton, and Mark, 1973.)

Possible functional effects on developmentally marked connections in the nervous system

If connection specifying markers have their expression modified by impulse activity in the peripheral nervous system, how much more likely this is in the higher reaches of the central nervous system? It is here that the developmentally marked space codes, so important for the faithful reconstruction of sensory maps in the brain and the maintenance of reliable interneuronal patterns of connection, begin to change their form. There is much convergance of synaptic input on to higher order neurones so that cortical cells in mammals, specially outside the primary projection areas for sensory pathways, can be found to respond to a wide variety of sensory stimuli, visual, auditory, tactile, and so on. Yet all these signals must have arrived on sensory pathways that peripherally, at least, maintained their topological relationships by the proposed gradient and specific molecular marker systems. As information is handed on from these systems to those showing less, or different kinds, of precision in synaptic connectivity the higher-order neurones must become less selective in the kind of marker substance they will accept in the formation of synapses.

Now, if the marker was very weak or in very low concentration in a pre-synaptic terminal, it may require impulse activity and transmission from the terminal to make its presence felt on the post-synaptic cell. This could be by injection of a specific trophic substance along with the transmitter or by the acceleration of synthesis of the specific marker proportional to impulse activity. If the marker had the action of suppressing transmission from converging synapses bearing different markers, just as it appears to have at neuromuscular junctions, we have a mechanism for prolonged synaptic change in favour of a used synapse and without visible structural alteration. Should this be the main mechanism for permanent modification of neuronal connections it is no wonder it has not yet been detected by anatomical or physiological methods. Anatomically, conventional electronmicroscopic techniques can make no distinction between functional and non-functional neuromuscular synapses. Therefore there is unlikely to be an obvious distinction between them if they exist in the brain. Physiologically, the expected change would be a diminution in effectiveness, not of those synaptic connections that are subject to use but of the unused convergent connections on to a common post-synaptic neurone. Most electrophysiological or biochemical theories (Eccles, 1965; Deutsch, 1971), have postulated, and searched for, a mechanism of increased transmitter effectiveness of frequently used connections. In fact, in the complex networks of real neurones, the overall functional effect of increasing effectiveness of one set of connections would be the same as diminishing the effectiveness of all the rest. An experiment designed to look for one mechanism, however, is quite likely to be blind to the other.

Learning therefore would consist of repressing transmission from many convergent synapses, leaving a neurone preferentially connected to one or a greatly reduced number of presynaptic pathways. The importance of the preceding developmental processes would be that the number of possible

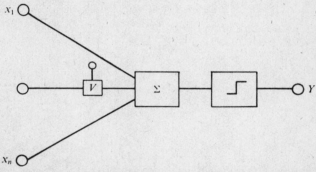

FIG. 14. An adaptive linear separation unit. Each input x is multiplied by a factor V and summed. If the total value exceeds a threshold there is an output at Y. If V is dependent in some way on the past history of use of each input terminal X, the device will show adaptive behaviour. In the present model of memory V, for a particular channel x tends to be reduced in value when other channels are active in the absence of an input at x. Unused pathways are therefore closed off. (From Uttley, 1970.)

interneuronal associations that could be developed through learning would depend upon the density of interneuronal connections set up by embryological mechanisms. This would provide the genetic basis for inherited behaviour patterns and the range of adaptability or intelligence. The individual would fulfil or squander his inheritance according to the patterns of interneuronal associations made within the limits of complexity set by the number of potentially available connections.

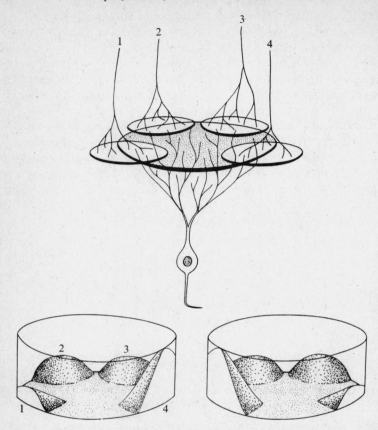

FIG. 15. As in Fig. 14 but in neuronal terms. Input fibres 1–4 make connections with a common neurone. The strength of connections is shown on the three-dimensional graphs below, with synaptic efficacy on the vertical axis and the area of connection corresponding to a horizontal section of the dendritic tree on the horizontal axis. On the left is the pattern of efficacy if fibre 4 is used more than the others, on the right the expected pattern if fibre 1 were the most frequently-used connection.

A physical system for a similar operation is known as a linear separation unit (Fig. 14). Each of a number of input terminals can sum to contribute to the output of the unit once a threshold value is exceeded. If the conductivity of the input pathways is modified by their history of use, then the output can come to signal the occurrence of particular spatial patterns of input. In the model corresponding to the repressed-synapse pattern detector, conductivity of each input pathway would remain constant when that pathway was used but would decrease when any other pathway was used. Frequent occurrence of a set of inputs, would progressively render other inputs less effective. Neurologically one would conceive of the output as representing a kind of motor behaviour, the inputs the set of all possible sensory stimuli that could contribute to this behaviour. Learning is the selection of those sensory patterns that are most often used by the competitive blocking of unused connections (Fig. 15). A theoretical treatment of related pattern detecting networks is given by Uttley (1970). Repressive systems for learning have previously been postulated by Young (1965) although of a slightly different kind to the one described here (Mark, 1970, 1973), and more recently by other theorists (Albus, 1971, Rosenzweig, Mollgaard, Daimond, and Bennett, 1972).

BIOLOGICAL CONSTRAINTS AND EVIDENCE FOR LEARNING BY SYNAPTIC REPRESSION

Are there enough connections produced in the development of the brain to make this scheme feasible? Undoubtedly there are. By quantitative electronmicroscopy it is possible to estimate the total number of morphologically recognizable synaptic contacts in a given volume of brain. In mammalian cortex the number is extraordinarily, almost astronomically large 10^{12} synapses cm^3. By light microscopy one can estimate the number of nerve-cell bodies in the same volume and by division one arrives at a statistical estimate of the number of synapses terminating on the average cell. In mammalian cortex this is of the order of 50 000 synapses per cell. On reaching this figure, Cragg (1967), who made the counts, immediately realized that this posed a serious physiological problem. Nerve cells act as integrators but how could integrating units each with an average of 50 000 inputs and 50 000 outputs possibly work?

One possibility is that each cell may make many connections with another, but the redundancy introduced this way is not likely to be more than 100 connections per cell and probably is less. Therefore, the figure for intercellular connectivity could come down to about 500. Even so, in the physical or mathematical model one thinks of at the moment, the digital computer, the corresponding connectivity of logical elements is 2. The brain certainly does not work like a computer but it would be much easier to understand if most of those synapses represented potential connections which could be eliminated by learning and if the real connectivity was very much lower. In the cerebral cortex (Scholl, 1956; Cragg, 1967) it is difficult on anatomical grounds to believe that every cell is not connected to every other one within reach. However, cortical neurones in the primary receiving areas at least show to a high degree the refinement of stimulus parameters for their excitation that is widely believed to be due to specific connectivity (Henry and Bishop, 1971).

Another neuroanatomist, Szentagothai, has estimated, informally, that the density of interconnections throughout the brain is such that one could trace a path via anatomical synaptic connections from any one neurone to any other one by passing through only five intermediate cells. Yet the physiological evidence of the specificity of connections in those parts of the brain where it can be studied shows that functional connections between the billion-odd neurones of the mammalian brain are by no means haphazard. Elsewhere Szentagothai (1967), speaking of the integrative interneurones of the spinal cord says 'almost every internuncial neurone inside the group of, for instance five neighbouring segments, may be connected with every other internuncial neurone'. Yet this is the region of the spinal cord containing neurones concerned with the regulation of muscle stretch and tension, the ordered relaxation of one muscle during the contraction of another, and the real nervous machinery for stepping and rhythmic locomotion (Jankowska and Lindstrom, 1972). All the detailed physiological work on the spinal cord has indicated that specific connection patterns, mediated by these interneurones, form the basis of these mechanisms (Eccles, 1964). A good body of circumstantial evidence can in fact be accumulated to suggest that functional connectivity between nerve cells is far more refined than is anatomical connectivity. For example, in the area of the first synapses from the sensory nerves of the face of the cat, the terminal arborizations contact cells which have long dendritic processes extending up and down the brain stem (Aström, 1953). Yet physiologically the response of these cells may be only elicited from a small peripheral receptive field and stimulation of afferent fibres from adjacent regions, the central process of which must surely cross the dendritic tree of the same cell, produces no effect (Wall and Taub, 1962; Darian-Smith, Proctor, and Ryan, 1963).

A more convincing demonstration that it is the relative effectiveness of central synapses that forms the boundaries of the receptive field of cells in the cat spinal cord comes from Merrill and Wall (1972). These spinal cord neurones are synaptically driven by sensory fibres from the skin, the natural stimulation of which will fire the cell from a restricted area that is easily defined. The primary sensory fibres enter the spinal cord over a fan of rootlets that may be separated from each other. It is not difficult to discover which rootlet takes the effective sensory fibres into the cord. However, having done this one may stimulate electrically adjacent rootlets bearing fibres from adjacent skin areas. Whereas natural stimulation of these fibres via the skin they supply evoked no cellular response, electrical stimulation of a whole bundle of them close to the cord does. Presumably these fibres end on the cell in question as synaptic terminals that are so ineffective either in transmitter release or post-synaptic membrane response that only synchronous activation of a large number of them can produce sufficient transmembrane current to fire the cell.

Other physiological experiments by Wall and Egger (1971) have given results that could be interpreted as indication of the presence of repressed synapses. In the thalamus of the rat, a synaptic relay station on the pathway from skin sense organs to the cerebral cortex, a very precise somatotopic map of the body surface can be revealed by moving a microelectrode through the region and correlating position of responses of single cells with the location of the skin area, the natural stimulation of which evokes their activity. Partial destruction of this pathway leads to a spread, beginning in about three days, of the somatotopic map into the region normally controlled by the damaged projections. This could either be due to new growth of pre-synaptic terminals on to nerve-cell bodies whose normal synapses had degenerated (Raisman, 1969), or to a recovery of function of existing previously repressed terminals due to removal of the dominant synapses.

If functional repression of convergent synapses is a normal mechanism of brain development it applies only to the last

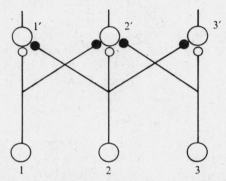

FIG. 16. Maintenance of the rank order among connecting sets of neurones by a mechanism of synaptic repression. Synaptic connections grow widely but repression of transmission from less well matched connections, i.e. those synapses onto neurone 2, from pre-synaptic neurones 1 and 3, restores the precision of functional connectivity.

fine details, which are organized on a scale easily visible by the electron microscope but right at the limits of resolution of the light microscope. It sounds quite reasonable that in the development of the topographically organized pathways there may be some overlap of synaptic connections between neurones from, say, adjacent areas of skin. The final development sorting out which commits the next neurone in the chain to responding to a particular set of primary nerve fibres could easily be dependent upon a competitive interaction between synapses of different peripheral origin for control of one neurone (Guillery, 1972) (Fig. 16). Connections eliminated by such a mechanism would not necessarily always degenerate and disappear. Microelectrode and electronmicroscopic analysis of skeletal muscle innervation in the axolotl has already given indications of the occurrence of competitive repression of synaptic transmission, from morphologically normal terminals as a normal mechanism in the formation of boundaries between segmental innervation territories (Cass *et al.*, 1973).

Other shreds of evidence for functionless connections come from studies of neuromuscular development. In the innervation of some involuntary muscle of the male sex organs, the vas deferens, nerve of normal ultrastructure and containing the transmitter substance, noradrenaline can be discovered several days before functional neuromuscular transmission in response to nerve stimulation will occur (Furness, McLean, and Burnstock, 1970). Certain bacterial toxins, botulinum toxin in particular, will render neuromuscular synapses inoperative by preventing transmitter release, but without degeneration in their ultrastructure (Thesleff, 1960).

The argument does not imply that the ordinary microscopic structure of the brain is functionally meaningless. Obviously other morphogenetic influences must be at work to produce the coarse structure of the brain, the rough general direction of growth of fibre tracts, the general topographic packing of fibres together according to their peripheral origin and the approximate number of nerve cells allowed to develop in any area. Older methods of differentially staining nerve fibres that are in the process of degeneration after being severed from the cell body, initially revealed this basic topographic organization of sensory and motor pathways. These maps in the brain, traced from sense organs to the cerebral cortex by following with light microscopy degenerating nerve fibres produced by carefully placed experimental damage to their axons, corresponded well to maps on a similar scale produced by electrical recording with crude electrodes that responded to the simultaneous stimulated activity of thousands of neurones in their vicinity.

When electrophysiological techniques improved to the point where the activity of single neurones could easily be recorded and anatomical techniques improved to allow the easy demonstration of single synapses by electron miscroscopy it was assumed that the anatomical and functional topographic maps would also coincide at this new level of resolution. In fact proof of such correspondence is lacking. It is assumed that every morphological synapse is in the same functionally effective state but there is no proof that this is so. It was not difficult to establish that chemical synaptic transmission is always associated with the characteristic profile of a synaptic terminal as seen by electronmicroscopy. To prove that the appearance of the profile may not always be associated with effective transmission from that very terminal could be difficult.

THE LINK BETWEEN SHORT-TERM AND LONG-TERM MODIFIABILITY

There remains to discuss the problem of how short-term changes of synaptic effectiveness may become translated into long-term structural modification by the proposed mechanism of synaptic repression. This is the question that plagues the neurophysiologist. One accepts that memory needs a structural change that involves new protein synthesis. How does information that comes into the nervous system in the form of discrete or identical nerve impulses, each one only 10^{-3}s long gain access to and then apparently redirect mechanisms for protein synthesis? Direct electrical links between the excitable membrane and macromolecular metabolism have been proposed but some more recent relevant evidence comes from analysis of the action of the drug ouabain on both memory formation and brain protein synthesis.

One obvious consequence of impulse activity is that the anterior of a nerve cell will gain sodium ions and lose potassium, because the metabolic pump which controls differential ion concentrations works so much more slowly than does the action potential mechanism. Furthermore the ion movements engendered by the pump can have direct effects on membrane potential and therefore electrical excitability (Ritchie and Straub, 1957; Baylor and Nicholls, 1969). These changes can last many minutes. Pump activity may be inhibited by ouabain (Glynn, 1964; Den Hertog and Ritchie, 1969) at concentrations that do not affect the impulse-carrying processes in any measurable way. This differential sensitivity enabled us to try the effect of ouabain directly on learning in chickens (Watts and Mark, 1971; and Chapter 4) leading to the finding that ouabain appeared to hasten the decline of short-term memory. This, and other experimental work, led to the hypothesis that there is a short-term memory process that is connected somehow to the metabolic recovery of recently active neurones and is independent of new protein synthesis. However, in the same experiment when permanent memory is examined, say three days after learning and ouabain treatment, ouabain is found to have been as effective as an inhibitor of protein synthesis in preventing long-term memory formation. This shows that whatever the mechanism of immediate action of ouabain on memory it also can prevent the process of consolidation into long-term store (Mark and Watts, 1971).

The action of ouabain on the enzymes responsible for its known action on sodium extrusion from nerve cells and on other enzyme systems for protein synthesis can be readily detected by biochemical techniques. On soluble extracts of homogenized brains it has no inhibitory effect on protein synthesis but does show an inhibition of the membrane enzyme responsible for sodium extrusion. However the brain in life is far from a homogenous soluble system, being comprised mainly of neuropil, that is the complex meshwork of cell processes, including synaptic terminals.

Careful breaking up of the brain and biochemical separation procedures can respect the intactness of membranes and produce a suspension of membrane-bound vesicles about 1m μm in diameter, many of which contain the organelles characteristic of synapses and a fragment of synaptic membrane of the broken post-synaptic cell. Such a preparation, containing resealed pre-synaptic terminals known as synaptosomes, and perhaps other membrane bound fragments, can extrude sodium in the normal way of nerve membranes and also synthesize protein from added amino acids. Ouabain, on this fraction, inhibits the activity of the sodium-pump enzymes and, in approximately the same proportion, the transport of amino acids into the vesicles and in consequence the amount of protein synthesized (Fig. 17); (Gibbs, Jeffrey, Austin and Mark, 1973).

Here, then, is a most intriguing connection between protein synthesis in small membrane-bound particles and the activity of the sodium pump. It suggests that protein synthesis in such a tissue may normally be limited by the availability of amino acids, perhaps only specific ones, and that their transport into the cell is linked in some way to the activity of the enzymes responsible for sodium extrusion. The exact nature of the link in biochemical terms is a matter for research but it is not difficult to imagine that a nerve cell that has accumulated sodium as a result of recent intense impulse activity and is in a state of accelerated sodium extrusion may also be accumulating amino acids or other as yet unspecified metabolic building blocks at a faster rate. This would lead to accelerated protein synthesis in recently active cells. No one knows the fate of protein synthesized by synaptosomal fractions of brain, but it may include a component involved in the intercellular recognition processes, and therefore influence synaptic connectivity

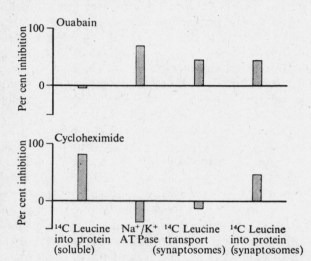

Fig. 17. The effect of ouabain and cycloheximide on protein synthesis and amino acid (^{14}C leucine) transport in chicken brain. A concentration of ouabain and cycloheximide giving equivalent inhibition of leucine incorporation into protein in the synaptosomal fraction has different effects on protein synthesis in soluble fractions, on the activity of enzymes responsible for sodium extrusion and on amino acid accumulation. Cycloheximide blocks protein synthesis by interference with the ribosomal mechanism and does not inhibit sodium/potassium ATPase, the sodium pump enzyme, or the accumulation of amino acid into the membrane-bound fragments of the synaptosomal fraction. Ouabain does not inhibit protein synthesis in soluble systems but does inhibit Na/KATPase and leucine accumulation in membrane-bound fragments. The inhibition of protein synthesis is proportional to the inhibition of amino acid transport, i.e. to the availability of substrate delivered by active membrane transport. (After Gibbs, Jeffrey, Austin, and Mark, 1973.)

by this mechanism. Ouabain also has been shown to have a strong inhibitory effect on protein synthesis in the intact brain, which might be expected as the amino acids delivered to the brain from the blood must be transported across two glial cell membranes and one neuronal cell membrane. In addition there may be direct effects of ouabain on protein synthesis within cells due to disorganization of the intracellular ionic conditions.

There is a great deal to be done in unravelling the connection between short- and long-term memory storage and ionic events and protein synthesis of nerve cells. At the moment there appears to be some relationship between these two sets of behavioural and biochemical observations. Both sets now need to be manipulated by similar experiments to see how far the correspondence goes. This can be done by broadening both approaches; using new and different learning tasks on whole animals (Rogers and Mark, 1973) and wider and more detailed biochemical analyses covering possible changes in neuronal RNA, and perhaps identification of the kind of protein produced by the nerve terminal fraction of homogenized brain. This method was used in the studies of antibiotics as inhibitors of long-term memory and now may be brought to bear on the possible mechanisms of action of the inhibitors of ionic metabolism and the initiation of memory.

A NEW HYPOTHESIS OF MEMORY

The whole working hypothesis can now be put together. In embryogenesis of topographically organized parts of the brain it is common for synaptic growth to be initially more widespread than the final functional pattern requires. Precision of connections depends upon competitive mechanisms acting to select the synaptic input best suited, on embryological grounds, to a given post-synaptic cell.

Comparison, of specific pre-synaptic marker substances, by recognition mechanisms in the post-synaptic cell is the method of selection and the method of operation is to suppress synaptic transmission from those terminals least well matched to the recipient neurones. On the input and output sides of the nervous system the scheme of embryological markers is very strong and leads to the orderly development of synaptic connections, without, or in spite of, functional interactions. It has never been proven that all anatomically recognizable synaptic processes can transmit. Perhaps even in precisely organized sensory pathways there are synapses retained that have suffered complete or partial competitive elimination.

At higher levels in the nervous system there is more interaction between sensory systems and accordingly post-synaptic cell recognition mechanisms must be modified to tolerate

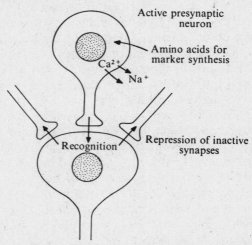

Fig. 18. Hypothesis of selection of synaptic connections according to use. Active neurones accumulate calcium and sodium, one or both of which will improve synaptic transmission for a short period. The increased activity of the Na+ pump leads to increased accumulation of amino acids or other organic molecules necessary for the synthesis of antibody-like marker proteins. The post-synaptic cell recognises the increased level of one marker and represses transmission from other cells bearing different markers.

many convergent synapses bearing weaker markers. Synaptic suppression in highly convergent systems can still occur if one set of terminals delivers a larger or more persistent dose of marker. Recognition of this by the post-synaptic element will set in train the operation of repression of synapses bearing other markers. In cells with very great convergence such changes in connectivity may be very small but, if a large number of interconnected cells are involved, small changes in each one could still produce a diametric change in the behaviour of the network to which they belonged.

Immediately following activity of one set of synapses their efficacy is increased, either by post-tetanic potentiation of transmitter release or by other mechanisms related to the ionic consequences of activity, perhaps the inexcitability of inhibitory interneurones. The restoration of Na : K ratios across the cell membrane by active metabolic transport of Na + is associated with an increase in transport into the cell of certain small organic molecules which contribute to the synthesis of specific marker proteins, leading to the initiation of the long-term changes (Fig. 18).

A mechanism of this kind is brought into operation during a critical period of an animal's early life for the final lining-up of neurones of the visual system in cats, frogs, and presumably other animals. At higher perceptual levels of the nervous system the same mechanism retains a flexibility, perhaps diminishing but effective throughout life, and continues to modify connectivity in neuronal networks, elminating unused pathways by competitive synaptic repression.

7 Conclusion

THE purpose of this book is to persuade the reader that it is sensible to view the ability of animals to store memories as a marginal extension into adult life of mechanisms that are responsible for the embryological development of the brain. The enduring modifiability of networks of neurones does not cut back across the functions of the network that were built in by well-protected developmental programmes but serves to change them only slightly according to the way they are most often used by the individual. This by itself is not an original thought (e.g. Sperry, 1962; Szilard, 1964; Jacobson, 1969; Gaze and Keating, 1971; Blakemore, 1972).

The difference between opinions previously expressed and the theory put forward here is that we now know just enough of the principles of development and synaptic transmission of neuromuscular connections to put up a reasonable hypothesis of a likely mechanism of synaptic selection in the central nervous system. From direct experiments with metabolic inhibitors of short-term memory we also have a notion of how this might be linked in with the impulse activity of nerve cells, on which the memory depends both for its registration and expression.

It is also argued that the discovery of the nature of the bio-chemical or physiological switch that ensures the permanent registration of memory is an easier scientific proposition than understanding the nature of the central nervous coding of environmental experience and the selection of appropriate behavioural responses. If the secrets of the patterns of brain activity subserving even very simple but modifiable fragments of behaviour were known, then it would be possible to find the precise location of the modifiable elements in the brain and find out how they work. However, by respecting the common features of neuronal metabolism and by the use of the most specific inhibitors of appropriate metabolic functions in well-designed experiments on learning, it may be possible to close the circle much sooner than expected and to know the kind of neuronal change responsible for memory storage long before much progress is made with the more difficult task of unravelling dynamic patterns of brain activity. This is a limited goal only in the sense that the discovery of the molecular nature of the gene was limited. Knowledge of the principles of modifiability of the brain will help in the next step of understanding perception, motivation, and the brain function underlying consciousness and self-awareness, just as knowledge of molecular genetics sets the pattern of thinking about the more complicated matters of cellular differentiation and embryological development.

The developmental attitude to learning is so reasonable on physiological grounds and is so satisfying from the point of the evolutionary emergence and significance of adaptive behaviour that it seems worth while investing a lot of scientific effort into trying to find out how much truth there is in these ideas. On the behavioural side one wonders to what extent is the theory of learning by synaptic repression compatible with psychological theory. Forgetting as interference and the primacy of early learning or imprinting are two matters that seem to fit with the idea, and perhaps others could be explored. Physiologically the techniques are mostly available now for dealing with the nervous system at its unit level, that of the nerve cell and synapse, and the central question in this hypothesis, the existence of a mechanism in adult brain for partial or complete repression of synaptic function, could certainly be answered. Should the mechanism exist, to what extent is it a normal part of development, can it be reversed, and does it intervene in the recovery of the brain from damage? In infancy, for example the phenomenon of audiogenic seizures in mice (Saunders, Bock, James, and Chen, 1972) could be due to synaptic de-repression in the cochlea nucleus, or, in old age, the slow recovery from neurological deficits produced by brain damage such as a stroke could be due to reawakening of long-repressed alternative pathways.

If the process is at the base of some kinds of neuronal plasticity of function, is it amplified or stabilized by other mechanisms to produce a rapid and reliable learning mechanism? A partially repressed synapse for example could induce morphological changes in the part of the post-synaptic cell membrane it contacts to complete the block of transmission. What of its biophysical mechanism? So far even at the neuromuscular junction this is quite unknown.

But what if all these ideas were quite wrong, as they certainly are in part, and learning turned out to have absolutely nothing whatsoever to do with embryological mechanisms? Would it be worth while in human or medical terms to continue with the search?

It would, of course, if only because the understanding of the brain is the only part of biology where the basic principles are still unknown. Most biomedical research in other fields is on fringe areas, the quasi-technological exploitation of known principles or the filling-in of quite small gaps in scientific knowledge by the use of experimental methods of ever-increasing cost and complexity. There is no challenge in hormone research beyond the technical. The molecular level of interactions is known in principle and there can be no really big surprises, which gives a confidence and a sense of direction to this research that is quite absent from any perceptive approach to the nervous system. To the most knowledgeable of scientists the brain is as dark and disquieting as were the cycle of the seasons and the mysteries of human birth, growth, and death to early man. We have some fragmentary principles, the nature of the nerve impulse and its transmission and cellular nature of the nervous system, but the cohesion of the whole thing, the undeniable unity of perception and response which emerges from the working brain has no scientific explanation even at a mechanistic level, let alone the problem of what to do about consciousness. The whole of human behaviour emerges from an organ almost entirely without relevant scientific description. Since human behaviour causes most of the trouble in the world now, the lack of understanding in an otherwise increasingly science-based society is serious.

Even if the idea of flexibility of brain function being based upon multiple potential connections made by repressed synapses turns out to be mainly correct this would be a small step in the complete physiological elucidation of memory.

In an intact animal this has a rapidity, reliability, and durability of action which can enormously exceed the changes that occur in any preparation that the neurophysiologist can put in a dish or impale with a microelectrode. From what property or combination of neuronal properties do these attributes emerge? Is there a unique biochemical process that can permanently and radically alter the function of a neurone or synapse? Is there a logical network property of electrical signalling between neurones in connection with each other that confers reliability upon a less reliable biochemical process? Do psychological concepts such as association and effect have any simple physiological reality? Is the idea of reinforcement critical for memory theories or is it, as some suspect, a concept which has emerged from the study of specific motivated behaviour and has no simple counterpart in the brain. These and many other specific questions must be answered in turn before we have any deep biological understanding of memory.

It is because these questions are so hard to attempt to answer at the moment that memory research tends to revert to the fantastic. Simple systems where one knows, or feels one knows, all the inputs and all the outputs and where one can measure information as discrete nerve impulses are more reassuring to manage. The results can be fascinating, but are not necessarily, or clearly, related to memory.

The idea of memory as a chain of amino acids or other molecules has a similar appeal. All the complexity of the real brain can then be taken on trust. It simply is a machine for reading peptide sequences and converting them into behaviour. It may be very complicated but that is only an engineering problem. Further research would consist in the decoding of further molecules, finding the difference between light and dark amino acid sequences or marvelling at how the chemistry of red memories differs from green and perhaps learning how to exploit this knowledge in the control or modi-fication of behaviour. There would be nothing more to it than a remapping of perceptual or behavioural concepts on to a molecular plane.

The alternative theory, that memory even if fundamentally chemical in nature is somehow an integral part of a be-havioural system and exists as a slight readjustment of func-tional connectivity that is only meaningful to the individual brain, is conceptually unsatisfying in the present state of neurophysiological knowledge. We have only the most sketchy outline of the neuronal systems involved in any behavioural act, we can only begin to comprehend the biochemical com-plexity of the mechanisms of interneuronal connectivity and it is completely impossible to guess which aspect of the pro-cess might be susceptible to changes produced by use. Quite rightly, from this angle, and with the hopes raised by molecu-lar theories, one finds references in general scientific litera-ture to 'the towering biological problem of memory'. Such sensationalism is not justified. Whether something towers or not depends on the vantage point of the observer. When the aims of memory research are set rather lower, some principles of brain physiology and development provide a viewpoint from which the feeling of hopelessness is not overwhelming and it becomes possible to plan for further understanding by application of the old scientific principles of hypothesis and experiment.

Of course, neural memory participates in the mechanisms of behaviour of all mobile animals and plays many different roles in each. It is no use trying to simplify the behavioural expression of all memory to the point where it can be treated as a physiological problem. Human memory, constrained as it is by the nature of the special receptor mechanisms of man and even by the cultural pressures of the societies in which we live may have nothing in common with memories in the brain of a rat, an octopus, or an ant, either in its information content or its powers to direct behaviour. The unity of outlook comes from the recognition of memory forma-tion as an extension of brain development, which makes it quite reasonable to suggest that within the limits set by em-bryological processes there may be a common selective mechanism represented widely in all animals and at all levels of their nervous systems, whereby frequently repeated patterns of nerve impulses can become incorporated into brain structure so that the reappearance of such patterns is guaranteed.

Bibliography

In order to make the text easier to read I have not given a full reference for each topic mentioned and I have kept citations down to one author, as far as possible. By using a bibliographic aid, such as Citation Index or the Index Medicus, one or two names can be made into a complete reference list that will quickly lead to important work not quoted here.

The outlines in Chapters 1–5 may be filled in by reference to the following:

CHAPTER 1

AIDLEY, D. J. (1971). *The physiology of excitable cells.* Cambridge University Press, London.

KATZ, B. (1966). *Nerve, muscle, and synapse.* McGraw-Hill, London.

MOUNTCASTLE, V. B. (ed). *Medical Physiology, Vol. II*, (12th edn.). C. V. Mosby, St. Louis.

CHAPTER 2

HILGARD, E. R. and BOWER, G. H. (1966). *Theories of learning*, (3rd edn.). Appleton-Century-Crofts, New York.

HINDE, R. A. (1966). *Animal behaviour: a synthesis of ethology and comparative psychology* (2nd edn.). McGraw-Hill, New York.

CHAPTER 3

GAZE, R. M. (1970). *The formation of nerve connections.* Academic Press, London.

JACOBSON, M. (1970). *Developmental neurobiology.* Holt, Rinehart and Winston, New York.

CHAPTER 4

BYRNE, W. L. (1970). *Molecular approaches to learning and memory.* Academic Press, New York.

GIBBS, M. E. and MARK, R. F. (1973). *Inhibition of memory formation.* Plenum Press, New York.

UNGAR, G. (1970). *Molecular mechanisms in memory and learning.* Plenum Press, New York.

CHAPTER 5

CRAGG, B. G. (1972). *Plasticity of synapses.* In *The structure and function of nervous tissue* (ed. G. H. Boune), vol. IV, pp. 1–66. Academic Press, New York.

KANDEL, E. R. and SPENCER, W. A. (1968). Cellular neurophysiological approaches in the study of learning. *Physiol. Rev.* **48**, 65–134.

In addition, interesting summaries of ideas in neurobiology can be found in:

QUARTON, G. C., MELNECHUK, T., and SCHMITT, F. O. (1967). *The neurosciences, a study program.* Rockefeller University Press, New York, and SCHMITT, F. O. (1970). *The neurosciences, second study program.* Rockefeller University Press, New York.

REFERENCES

A CORRESPONDENT. (1972). Why do brain cells synthesize protein. *Nature New Biol.* **230**, 100.

ADAIR, L. B., WILSON, J. E., and GLASSMAN, E. (1968). Brain function and macromolecules. IV. Uridine incorporation into polysomes of mouse brain during different behavioral experiences. *Proc. Natn. Acad. Sci. U.S.A.* **61**, 917–22.

AGRANOFF, B. W., DAVIS, R. E., and BRINK, J. J. (1966). Chemical studies on memory fixation in goldfish. *Brain Res.* **1**, 303–9.

AGRANOFF, B. W., DAVIS, R. E., CASOLA, L., and LIM, R. (1967). Actinomycin D blocks formation of memory of shock avoidance in goldfish. *Science* **158**, 1600–1.

AGUILAR, C. E., BISBY, M. A., and DIAMOND, J. (1972). Impulses and the transfer of trophic factors in nerves. *J. Physiol.* (July), 26P.

AKERT, K. (1949). Der visuelle Greifreflex. *Helv. physiol. pharmacol. Acta.* **7**, 112–34.

ALBUS, J. S. (1971). A theory of cerebellar function. *Math. Biosci.* **10**, 25–61.

ASTRÖM, K. E. (1953). On the central course of the afferent fibres in the trigeminal, facial glossopharyngeal and vagal nerves and their nuclei in the mouse. *Acta. physiol. Scand.* **29** Suppl. **106**, 209–320.

ATTARDI, D. G. and SPERRY, R. W. (1963). Preferential selection of central pathways by regenerating optic fibres. *Expt Neurol.* **7**, 46–64.

BABICH, F. R., JACOBSON, A. L., BUBASH, S., and JACOBSON, A. (1965). Transfer of a response to naïve rats by injection of ribonucleic acid extracted from trained rats. *Science* **149**, 656–7.

BAKER, R. E. and JACOBSON, M. (1970). Development of reflexes from skin grafts in *Rana pipiens*: influence of size and position of grafts. *Develop. Biol.* **22**, 476–94.

BARLOW, H. B. and PETTIGREW, J. D. (1971). Lack of specificity of neurones in the visual cortex of young kittens. *J. Physiol.* **218**, 98–100P.

BARONDES, S. H. (1970). Cerebral protein synthesis inhibitors block long-term memory. *Internat. Rev. Neurobiol.* **12**, 177–205.

BARONDES, S. H. and COHEN, H. D. (1966). Puromycin effect on successive phases of memory storage. *Science* **151**, 594–5.

BARONDES, S. H. and COHEN, H. D. (1967). Comparative effects of cyclo-heximide and puromycin on cerebral protein synthesis and consolidation of memory in mice. *Brain Res.* **4**, 44–51.

BARONDES, S. H. and COHEN, H. D. (1968). Arousal and the conversion of short-term to long-term memory. *Proc. Natn. Acad. Sci. U.S.A.* **61**, 923–9.

BARONDES, S. H. and JARVIK, M. E. (1964). The influence of actinomycin D on brain RNA synthesis and memory. *J. Neurochem.*, **11**, 187–95.

BATESON, P. P. G. (1970). Are they really products of learning? In *Short-term changes in neural activity and behaviour* (eds. G. Horn and R. A. Hinde), pp. 553–64. Cambridge University Press, London.

BATESON, P. P. G., HORN, G., and ROSE, S. P. R. (1972). Effects of early experience on regional incorporation of precursors into RNA and protein in the chick brain. *Brain Res.* **39**, 449–65.

BAYLOR, D. A. and NICHOLLS, J. G. (1969). After-effects of nerve impulses on signalling in the central nervous system of the leech, *J. Physiol.* **203**, 571–89.

BAYLOR, D. A. and NICHOLLS, J. G. (1971). Patterns of regeneration between individual nerve cells in the central nervous system of the leech. *Nature* **232**, 268–9.

BEACH, F. A. (1955). The descent of instinct. *Psychol. Rev.* **62**, 401–10.

BERLYNE, D. E. (1960). *Conflict, arousal and curiosity*, p. 174. McGraw-Hill, New York.

BERNSTEIN, J. J. and GELDRED, J. B. (1970). Regeneration of the long spinal tracts in the goldfish. *Brain Res.* **20**, 33–8.

BINDMAN, L. J. and BOISACQ-SCHEPPENS (1966). Persistent changes in the rate of firing of single spontaneously active cells in the rat produced by peripheral stimulation. *J. Physiol.* **185**, 14–17P.

BINDMAN, L. J., LIPPOLD, O. C. J., and REDFEARN, J. W. T. (1962). Long-lasting changes in the level of electrical activity of the cerebral cortex produced by polarizing currents. *Nature* **196**, 584–5.

BLACK, I. B., BLOOM, F. E., HENDRY, I. A., and IVERSEN, L. L. (1971). Growth and development of a sympathetic ganglion: maturation of transmitter enzymes and synapse formation in the mouse superior cervical ganglion. *J. Physiol.* **215**, 24–5P.

BLAKEMORE, C. (1972). Strategies of adaptive modification in the kitten's visual cortex. *Paper presented to the VIth International Meeting of Neurobiologists, St. Catherine's College, Oxford.*

BLAKEMORE, C. and COOPER, G. F. (1970). Development of the brain depends on the visual environment. *Nature* **228**, 477–8.

BLISS, T. V. P., BURNS, B. D., and UTTLEY, A. M. (1968). Factors affecting the conductivity of pathways in the cerebral cortex. *J. Physiol.* **195**, 339–67.

BLISS, T. V. P. and LØMO, T. (1970). Plasticity in a monosynaptic cortical pathway. *J. Physiol.* **207**, 61P.

BLOUGH, D. S. (1958). A method for obtaining pyschophysical thresholds from the pigeon. *J. exp. Anal. Behav.* **1**, 31–43.

BOISACQ-SCHEPPENS, N. (1968). Comparaison des effets prolongés de la stimulation somatique sur la fréquence de décharge spontanée de neurones corticaux chez le rat anesthesié ou non. *Archs. Internat. Physiol. Biochem.* **76**, 562–4.

BOLLES, R. C. (1972). Reinforcement expectancy and learning. *Psychol. Rev.* **79**, 394–409.

BOOTH, D. A. (1967). Vertebrate brain ribonucleic acids and memory retention. *Psychol. Bull.* **68**, 149–77.

BRINDLEY, G. S. (1967). The classification of modifiable synapses and their use in models for conditioning. *Proc. Roy. Soc. B* **168**, 361–76.

BRINDLEY, G. S. (1969). Nerve-net models of plausible size that perform many simple learning tasks. *Proc. Roy. Soc. B* **174**, 173–91.

BRINDLEY, G. S. (1970). Chemical mnemonology (book review). *Nature* **228**, 583.

BROADBENT, D. E. (1970). Psychological aspects of short-term and long-term memory. *Proc. Roy. Soc. B* **175**, 333–50.

BURNS, B. D. (1968). *The uncertain nervous system.* Edward Arnold Ltd. London.

BYRNE, W. L. (1970). *Molecular approaches to learning and memory.* Academic Press, New York.

BYRNE, W. L. (and 22 other authors) (1966). Memory transfer. *Science* **153**, 658.

CAJAL, S. RAMON (1955). *Histologie du système nerveux de l'homme et des vertebres,* Vols. *I* and *II.* Maloine, Paris, 1911; *Reprinted Instituto Cajal, Madrid.*

CAJAL, S. RAMON (1959). *Degeneration and regeneration of the nervous system* (translated by R. M. May). Hafner, New York.

CAJAL, S. RAMON, (1960). *Studies on vertebrate neurogenesis* (revised and translated by L. Guth). Charles C. Thomas, Springfield, Illinois.

CASS, D. T. and MARK, R. F. (1972). Microelectrode investigation of reinnervation of skeletal muscles in the axolotl (*Ambystoma mexicanum*) *Proc. Austral. Physiol. pharm. Soc.* **3**, 33–4.

CASS, D. T., SUTTON, T. J., and MARK, R. F. (1973). Competition between nerves for functional connections with axolotl muscles. *Nature* (in the press).

CHERKIN, A. (1966). Toward a quantitative view of the engram. *Proc. Natn. Acad. Sci. U.S.A.* **55**, 88–91.

CHILD, C. M. (1941). *Patterns and problems of development.* University of Chicago Press, Chicago.

CHOMSKY, N. (1967). The formal nature of language. In *Biological basis of language* (ed. E. H. Lenneberg), pp. 397–442. Wiley, London.

CRAGG, B. G. (1967). The density of synapses and neurones in the motor and visual areas of the cerebral cortex. *J. Anat.* **101**, 639–54.

CRAGG, B. G. (1972). Plasticity of synapses. In *The Structure and function of nervous tissue* (ed. G. H. Bourne), vol. 4, pp. 1–60. Academic Press, New York.

CRAIK, F. I. M. and LOCKHART, R. S. (1972). Levels of processing: a framework for memory research. *J. verb. Learn. verb. Behav.* **11**, 671–84.

CRICK, F. (1970). Diffusion in embryogenesis. *Nature* **225**, 420–22.

CRONLY-DILLON, J. R. (1968). Pattern of retinotectal connections after retinal regeneration. *J. Neurophysiol.* **31**, 410–18.

DALE, H. H. (1934). Pharmacology and nerve endings. *Proc. Roy. Soc. Medecine* **28**, 319–332.

DANIELS, D. (1971). Effect of actinomycin D on memory and brain RNA synthesis in an appetitive learning task. *Nature* **231**, 395–7.

DARIAN-SMITH, I., PROCTOR, R., and RYAN, R. D. (1963). A single-neurone investigation of somatotopic organization within the cat's trigeminal brain stem nuclei. *J. Physiol.* **168**, 147–57.

DEN HERTOG, A. and RITCHIE, J. M. (1969). A comparison of the effect of temperature, metabolic inhibitors and of ouabain on the electrogenic components of the sodium-pump in mammalian non-myelinated nerve fibres. *J. Physiol.* **204**, 523–38.

DEUTSCH, J. A. (1971). The cholinergic synapse and the site of memory. *Science* **174**, 788–94.

DEWS, P. B. and WIESEL, T. N. (1970). Consequences of monocular deprivation on visual behaviour in kittens. *J. Physiol.* **206**, 437–55.

DYAL, J. A. (1971). Transfer of behavioural bias and learning enhancement: a critique of specificity experiments. In *Biology of memory* (ed. G. Adam), pp. 145–59. Plenum Press, New York.

ECCLES, J. C. (1964). *The physiology of synapses.* Springer-Verlag, Berlin.

ECCLES, J. C. (1969). *The inhibitory pathways of the central nervous system,* Liverpool University Press, Liverpool.

ECCLES, J. C. (and others) (1965). Possible ways in which synaptic mechanisms participate in learning, remembering, and forgetting. In *The anatomy of memory* (ed. D. P. Kimble), pp. 12–87. Science and Behaviour Books, Palo Alto.

ECCLES, J. C., ITO, M., and SZENTAGOTHAI, J. (1967). *The cerebellum as a neuronal machine* (p. 276, disfacilitation). Springer Verlag, Berlin.

EDWARDS, J. J. and PALKA, J. (1971). Delayed formation of central contacts by insect sensory cells. *Science* **172**, 591–4.

EISENSTEIN, E. M. and COHEN, M. J. (1965). Learning in isolated prothoracic ganglion, *Animal Behav.* **13**, 104–8.

ELAZAR, Z. and ADEY, W. R. (1967). Electroencephalic correlates of learning in subcortical and cortical structures. *Electroenceph. clin. Neurophysiol.* **23**, 306–17.

ERLICH, P. (1956). *The collected papers of Paul Erlich* (eds. F. Himmelweit, M. Marquardt, and H. H. Dale), 3 vols. Pergamon Press, London.

FAREL, P. B. and BUERGER, A. A. (1972). Instrumental conditioning of leg position in chronic spinal frog: before and after sciatic section. *Brain Res.* **47**, 345–51.

FELDMAN, J. D., GAZE, R. M., and KEATING, M. J. (1971). The effect on intertectal connexions of rearing *Xenopus laevis* in total darkness. *J. Physiol.* **212**, 44–5P.

FILLENZ, M. (1972). Hypothesis for a neuronal mechanism involved in memory. *Nature* **238**, 41–3.

FJERDINGSTAD, E. V. (1969). Chemical transfer of alternation training in the Skinner box. *Scand. J. Psychol.* **10**, 220–4.

FLEXNER, L. B. and FLEXNER, J. B. (1968). Intra-cerebral saline: effect on memory of trained mice treated with puromycin. *Science* **159**, 330–1.

FRANK, B., STEIN, D. G., and ROSEN, J. (1970). Inter-animal 'memory' transfer: results from brain and liver homogenates. *Science* **169**, 399–402.

FURNESS, J. B., McLEAN, J. R., and BURNSTOCK, G. (1970). Distribution of adrenergic nerves and changes in neuromuscular transmission in the mouse vas deferens during postnatal development, *Develop. Biol.* **21**, 491–505.

GAGE, P. W. and HUBBARD, J. I. (1966). An investigation of post-tetanic potentiation of end plate potentials at a mammalian neuromuscular junction. *J. Physiol.* **184**, 353–75.

GAITO, J. (1971). *DNA complex and adaptive behaviour.* Prentice-Hall, Englewood Cliffs, New Jersey.

GAITO, J. (1972). *Macromolecules and behaviour* (2nd edn.). Appleton-Century-Crofts, New York.

GARDNER-MEDWIN, A. R. (1969). Modifiable synapses necessary for learning. *Nature* **223**, 916–19.

GARTSIDE, I. B. (1968a). Mechanisms of sustained increases in firing rate of neurones in the rat cerebral cortex after polarization: reverberating circuits or modification of synaptic conductance. *Nature* **220**, 382–83.

GARTSIDE, I. B. (1968b). Mechanisms of sustained increases of firing rate of neurones in the rat cerebral cortex after polarization: role of protein synthesis. *Nature* **220**, 383–4.

GAZE, R. M. (1958). The representation of the retina on the optic lobe of the frog. *Quart. J. Exp. Physiol.* **43**, 209–14.

GAZE, R. M. (1960). Regeneration of the optic nerve in amphibia. *Internat. Rev. Neurobiol.* **2**, 1–40.

GAZE, R. M., CHUNG, S. H., and KEATING, M. J. (1972). Development of the retinotectal projection in *Xenopus*. *Nature New Biol.* **236**, 133–5.

GAZE, R. M. and JACOBSON, M. (1962). The projection of the binocular visual field on the optic tecta of the frog. *Quart. J. Exp. Physiol.* **47**, 273–80.

GAZE, R. M., JACOBSON, M., and SZEKELY, G. (1963). The retino-tectal projection in *Xenopus* with compound eyes. *J. Physiol.* **165**, 484–99.

GAZE, R. M., JACOBSON, M., and SZEKELY, G. (1965). On the formation of connexions by compound eyes in *Xenopus*. *J. Physiol.* **176**, 409–17.

GAZE, R. M. and KEATING, M. J. (1971). Functional control of nerve fibre connections. In *Biology of memory* (ed. G. Adam), pp. 37–44.

GAZE, R. M., KEATING, M. J., SZEKELY, G., and BEAZLEY, L. (1970). Binocular interaction in the formation of specific intertectal neuronal connexions. *Proc. Roy. Soc. B.* **175**, 107–47.

GAZE, R. M. and SHARMA, S. C. (1970). Axial differences in the reinnervation of the goldfish optic tectum by regenerating optic nerve fibres. *Expmtl. Brain. Res.* **10**, 171–81.

GIBBS, M. E., JEFFREY, P. L., AUSTIN, L., and MARK, R. F. (1973). Biochemical aspects of drug inhibition of memory formation in chickens. *Pharmacol. Biochem. Behav.* (in press).

GIBBS, M. E. and MARK, R. F. (1973). *Inhibition of memory formation.* Plenum Press, New York.

GLASSMAN, E. (1969). The biochemistry of learning: an evaluation of the role of RNA and protein. *Ann. Rev. Biochem.* **38**, 605–46.

GLYNN, I. M. (1964). The action of cardiac glycosides on ion movements. *Pharmac. Rev.* **16**, 381–407.

GRAFSTEIN, B. and BURGEN, A. S. V. (1964). Pattern of optic nerve connections following retinal regeneration. *Prog. Brain Res.* **6**, 126–38.

GRIFFITH, J. S. (1966). A theory of the nature of memory. *Nature* **211**, 1160–3.

GRIMM, L. M. (1971). An evaluation of myotypic respecification in axolotls. *J. Expmtl. Zool.* **178**, 479–96.

GUILLERY, R. W. (1972). Binocular competition in the control of geniculate cell growth, *J. comp. Neurol.* **144**, 117–30.

GUTH, L. and BERNSTEIN, J. J. (1961). Selectivity in the re-establishment of synapses in the superior cervical ganglion of the cat. *Expmtl. Neurol.* **4**, 59–69.

GUTHRIE, E. R. (1959). Association by contiguity. In *Psychology: a study of a science* (ed. S. Koch), vol. 2, pp. 158–95. McGraw-Hill, New York.

VAN HARREVELD, A. (1966). *Brain tissue electrolytes.* Butterworths, London.

HARRISON, R. G. (1910). The outgrowth of the nerve fiber as a mode of protoplasmic movement. *J. Expmtl. Zool.* **9**, 787–846.

HARRISON, R. G. (1935). The origin and development of the nervous system studied by the methods of experimental embryology. *The Croonian Lecture. Proc. Roy. Soc. B.* **118**, 155–96.

HEBB, D. O. (1949). *Organization of behaviour.* Ch. 4. John Wiley and Sons, New York.

HEBB, D. O. (1958). Alice in wonderland or pyschology among the biological sciences. In *Biological and biochemical bases of behaviour* (eds. H. F. Harlow. and C. N. Woolsey), pp. 451–67. University of Wisconsin Press, Madison.

HENRY, G. H. and BISHOP, P. O. (1971). Simple cells of the striate cortex. In *Contributions to sensory physiology* (ed. W. D. Neff). Academic Press, New York.

HIBBARD, E. (1964). Selective innervation and reciprocal functional suppression from grafted extra labyrinths in amphibians. *Expmtl. Neurol.* **10**, 271–83.

HIBBARD, E. (1965). Orientation and directed growth of cell axons from duplicated vestibular nerve roots. *Expmtl. Neurol.* **13**, 289–301.

HILGARD, E. R. and BOWER, G. H. (1966). *Theories of learning.* Appleton-Century-Crofts, New York.

HIRSCH, H. V. B. (1972). Visual perception in cats after environmental surgery. *Expmtl. Brain Res.* **15**, 405–23.

HIRSCH, H. V. B. and SPINELLI, D. N. (1971). Modification of the distribution of receptive field orientation in cats by selective visual exposure during development. *Expmtl. Brain Res.* **13**, 509–27.

HODGKIN, A. L. (1964). *The conduction of the nervous impulse.* Liverpool University Press, Liverpool.

HORN, A. L. D. and HORN, G. (1969). Modification of leg flexion in response to repeated stimulation in a spinal amphibian (*Xenopus mullerei*). *Animal Behav.* **17**, 618–23.

HORN, G. (1970). Changes in neuronal activity and their relationship to behaviour. In *Short-term changes in neural activity and behaviour* (eds. G. Horn and R. A. Hinde), pp. 567–606. Cambridge University Press, London.

HORN, G. and HINDE, R. A. (eds.) (1970). *Short-term changes in neural activity and behaviour.* Cambridge University Press, Cambridge.

HORRIDGE, G. A. (1962). The learning of leg position by the ventral nerve cord in headless insects. *Proc. Roy. Soc. B.* **157**, 33–52.

HORRIDGE, G. A. (1967). Five types of memory in crab eye responses. In *Physiological and biochemical aspects of nervous integration* (ed. F. D. Carlson), pp. 245–64. Prentice-Hall, New Jersey.

HORRIDGE, G. A. (1968). *Interneurons*, Ch. 4. W. H. Freeman and Company, San Francisco.

HORRIDGE, G. A. and MEINERTZHAGEN, I. A. (1970). The accuracy of the patterns of connections of the first and second order neurons of the visual system of *Calliphora*. *Proc. Roy. Soc. B.* **175**, 69–82.

HOYLE, G. (1965). Neurophysiological studies on 'learning' in headless insects. In *Physiology of the insect central nervous system* (ed. J. Treheren). Academic Press, New York.

HUBEL, D. H. and WIESEL, T. N. (1959). Receptive fields of single neurons in the cat's striate cortex. *J. Physiol.* **148**, 574–91.

HUBEL, D. H. and WIESEL, T. N. (1962). Receptive fields binocular interaction and functional architecture in the cat's visual cortex. *J. Physiol.* **160**, 106–54.

HUBEL, D. H. and WIESEL, T. N. (1963). Receptive fields of cells in the striate cortex of very young visually inexperienced kittens. *J. Neurophysiol.* **26**, 994–1002.

HUBEL, D. H. and WIESEL, T. N. (1965). Binocular interaction in striate cortex of kittens reared with artificial squint. *J. Neurophysiol.* **28**, 1041–59.

HUBEL, D. H. and WIESEL, T. N. (1970). The period of susceptibility to the physiological effects of unilateral eye closure in kittens. *J. Physiol.* **206**, 419–36.

HUGHES, A. F. W. (1968). *Aspects of neural ontogeny.* Academic Press, London.

VON HUNGEN, K. (1971). Competitive hybridization with brain RNA fails to confirm new RNA induced by learning. *Nature* **229**, 114–15.

HYDÉN, H. (1943). Protein metabolism in the nerve cell during growth and function. *Acta. Physiol. Scand.* **6**, *Suppl.* 17, 1–136.

HYDÉN, H. and EGYHÁZI, E. (1962). Nuclear RNA changes of nerve cells during a learning experiment in rats. *Proc. Natn. Acad. Sci. U.S.A.* **48**, 1366–73.

HYDÉN, H. and EGYHÁZI, E. (1964). Changes in RNA content and base composition in cortical neurones of rats in a learning experiment involving transfer of handedness. *Proc. Nat. Acad. Sci. U.S.A.* **52**, 1030–5.

HYDÉN, H. and LANGE, P. W. (1968). Microelectrophonetic determinations of protein and protein synthesis in the 10^{-9} to 10^{-7} gram range. *J. Chromatogr.* **35**, 336–51.

HYDÉN, H. and LANGE, R. W. (1970). S100 protein correlation with behaviour. *Proc. Nat. Acad. Sci. U.S.A.* **67**, 1959–66.

JACOBSON, M. (1968a). Development of neuronal specificity in retinal ganglion cells of *Xenopus*. *Develop. Biol.* **17**, 202–18.

JACOBSON, M. (1968b). Cessation of DNA synthesis in retinal ganglion cells correlated with the time of specification of their central connections. *Develop. Biol.* **17**, 219–32.

JACOBSON, M. (1969). Development of specific neuronal connections. *Science* **163**, 543–7.

JACOBSON, M. (1971). Absence of adaptive modification in developing retinotectal connections in frogs after visual deprivation or disparate stimulation of the eyes. *Proc. Nat. Acad. Sci. U.S.A.* **68**, 528–32.

JACOBSON, M. and BAKER, R. E. (1969). Development of neuronal connections with skin grafts in frogs: behavioural and electrophysiological studies. *J. Comp. Neurol.* **137**, 121–42.

JAMES, W. (1890). *The principles of psychology*, vols. I and II. Macmillan, London.

JANKOWSKA, E. and LINDSTRÖM, S. (1972). Morphology of interneurones mediating Ia reciprocal inhibition of motoneurones in the spinal cord of the cat. *J. Physiol.* **226**, 805–23.

JANSEN, J. K. S. and NICHOLLS, J. G. (1972). Regeneration of changes in synaptic connections between individual nerve cells in the central nervous system of the leech. *Proc. Nat. Acad. Sci. U.S.A.* **69**, 636–9.

JOHN, E. R. (1967). *Mechanisms of memory*. Academic Press, New York.

KAPPERS, C. U. ARIENS, HUBER, G. C., and CROSBY (1960). *The comparative anatomy of the nervous system of vertebrates including man*. 3 vols. Reprinted by Hafner, New York.

KANDEL, E. R. and SPENCER, W. A. (1968). Cellular neurophysiological approaches in the study of learning. *Physiol. Rev.* **48**, 65–134.

KANDEL, E. R. and TAUC, L. (1965). Heterosynaptic facilitation in neurones of the abdominal ganglion of *Aplysia depilans*. *J. Physiol.* **181**, 1–27.

KATZ, B. (1969). *The release of neural transmitter substances*. Liverpool University Press, Liverpool.

KATZ, B. and MILEDI, R. (1965). The effect of calcium on acetylcholine release from motor nerve terminals. *Proc. Roy. Soc. B.* **161**, 496–503.

KATZ, B. and MILEDI, R. (1968). The role of calcium in neuromuscular facilitation. *J. Physiol.* **195**, 481–92.

KATZ, B. and MILEDI, R. (1970). Further study of the role of calcium in synaptic transmission. *J. Physiol.* **207**, 789–801.

KATZ, J. J. and HALSTEAD, W. C. (1950). Protein organization and mental function. *Comp. Psychol. Monographs.* **20**, 1–38.

KEATING, M. J. (1968). Functional interaction in the development of specific connections. *J. Physiol.* **198**, 75–7P.

KEATING, M. J. and GAZE, R. M. (1970). The ipsilateral retinotectal pathways in the frog. *Quart. J. Expmtl. Physiol.* **55**, 284–92.

KETY, S. S. (1972). Brain catecholamines affective states and memory. In *The chemistry of mood motivation and behaviour* (ed. J. McGaugh), pp. 65–80. Plenum Press, New York.

KEYNES, R. D. and RITCHIE, J. M. (1965). The movement of labelled ions in mammalian non-myelinated nerve fibres. *J. Physiol.* **179**, 333–67.

KOCH, R. (1880). *Investigations into the etiology of traumatic infectious diseases* (Translated by W. Watson Cheyne). The New Sydenham Society, London.

KRECH, D. (1972). In *The chemistry of mood motivation and behaviour; advances in behavioural biology*, vol. 4 (ed. J. C. McGough), pp. 217–23. Plenum Press, New York.

KRECH, D., ROSENZWEIG, M. R., and BENNETT, E. L. (1960). Effects of environmental complexity and training on brain chemistry. *J. Comp. Physiol. Psychol.* **53**, 509–19.

KUFFLER, S. W. and NICHOLLS, J. G. (1966). The physiology of neuroglial cells, *Ergeb. Physiol.* **57**, 1–90.

KUNO, M., MIYAHARA, J. T., and WEAKLY, J. N. (1970). Post-tetanic hyperpolarization produced by an electrogenic pump in dorsal spinocerebellar tract neurones of the cat. *J. Physiol.* **210**, 839–55.

LAJTHA, A. (1970). *Protein metabolism in the nervous system.* Plenum Press, New York.

LANDMESSER, L. and PILAR, G. (1970). Selective reinnervation of two cell populations in the adult pigeon ciliary ganglion. *J. Physiol.* **211**, 203–16.

LANGLEY, J. N. (1895). Note of regeneration of pre-ganglionic fibres of the sympathetic. *J. Physiol.* **28**, 280–4.

LASHLEY, K. S. (1950). In *Search of the engram.* In *Physiological mechanisms in animal behaviour*, *Soc. Exp. Biol. Symp. No.* 4, p. 454–82. Academic Press, New York.

LASHLEY, K. S. (1960). *The neuropsychology of Lashley* (eds. F. A. Beach. D. O. Hebb, C. T. Morgan, and H. W. Nissen). McGraw-Hill, New York.

LENNEBERG, E. H. (1967). *Biological foundations of language.* Wiley, New York.

LICKEY, M. E. (1969). Seasonal modulation and non-24-hour entrainment of a circadian rhythm in a single neuron. *J. Comp. Physiol. Psychol.* **68**, 9–17.

LILIEN, J. (1969). Toward a molecular explanation for specific cell adhesion. *Current Topics in developmental Biology* **4**, 169–95.

LLOYD, D. P. C. (1949). Post-tetanic potentiation of response in monosynaptic reflex pathways of the spinal cord. *J. Gen. Physiol.* **33**, 147–70.

LØMO, T. (1971). Potentiation of monosynaptic EPSPs in the perforant path-dentate granule cell synapse, *Expmtl. Brain Res.* **12**, 46–63.

LONGUET-HIGGINS, H. C., WILLSHAW, D. J., and BUNEMAN, O. P. (1970). Theories of associative recall. *Quart. Rev. Biophys.* **3**, 223–44.

LUCO, J. V. and ARANDA, L. C. (1964). An electrical correlate to the process of learning. Experiments in *Blatta orientalis. Nature* **201**, 1330–1331.

LUKOWIAK, K. and JACKLETT, J. W. (1972–3). Habituation and dishabituation: interactions between peripheral and central nervous system in *Aplysia. Science* **178**, 1306–8.

MACHLUS, B. and GAITO, J. (1969). Successive competition hybridization to detect RNA species in a shock avoidance task. *Nature* **222**, 573–4.

MALLART, A. and MARTIN, A. R. (1967). An analysis of facilitation of transmitter release on the neuromuscular junction of the frog. *J. Physiol.* **193**, 679–94.

MARK, R. F. (1965). Fin movement after regeneration of neuromuscular connections: an investigation of myotypic specificity. *Expmtl. Neurol.* **12**, 292–302.

MARK, R. F. (1969). Matching muscles and motoneurones. A review of some experiments on motor nerve regeneration. *Brain Res.* **14**, 245–54.

MARK, R. F. (1970). Chemospecific synaptic repression as a possible memory store. *Nature* **225**, 178–9.

MARK, R. F. (1973). Cellular mechanisms of neural memory. *Rep. Austral. Acad. Sci.* No. 16.

MARK, R. F. and FELDMAN, J. (1972). Binocular interaction in the development of optokinetic reflexes in tadpoles of *Xenopus laevis*. *Invest. Ophthal.* **11**, 402–10.

MARK, R. F. and MAROTTE, L. R. (1972). The mechanism of selective reinnervation of fish eye muscles. III. Functional, electrophysiological and anatomical analysis of recovery from section of the IIIrd and IVth nerves. *Brain Res.* **46**, 131–48.

MARK, R. F., MAROTTE, L. R., and MART, P. E. (1972). The mechanism of selective reinnervation of fish eye muscles. IV. Identification of repressed synapses. *Brain Res.* **46**, 149–57.

MARK, R. F., PEER, O., and STEINER, J. (1973). Integrative functions of the midbrain commissures in fish. *Expmtl. Neurol.* **39**, 140–156.

MARK, R. F. and WATTS, M. E. (1971). Drug inhibitions of memory formation in chickens. I. Long-term memory. *Proc. Roy. Soc.* B **178**, 439–54.

MAROTTE, L. R. and MARK, R. F. (1970a). The mechanism of selective reinnervation of fish eye muscle. I. Evidence from muscle function during recovery. *Brain Res.* **19**, 41–51.

MAROTTE, L. R. and MARK, R. F. (1970b). The mechanism of selective reinnervation of fish eye muscle. II. Evidence from electronmicroscopy of nerve endings. *Brain Res.* **19**, 53–69.

MARR, D. (1969). A theory of cerebellar cortex. *J. Physiol.* **202**, 437–70.

MARR, D. (1970). A theory for the cerebral neocortex, *Proc. Roy. Soc.* B **176**, 161–234.

MARR, D. (1971). Simple memory: a theory for archicortex, 262. *Phil. Trans. Roy. Soc.* B **262**, 23–81.

MART, P. E. and MARK, R. F. (1972). Ultrastructure of neuromuscular junctions during reinnervation of fast and slow muscle fibres in the axolotl. Paper presented at I.U.P.S. Regional Meeting, Sydney.

MATURANA, H. R., LETTVIN, J. Y., McCULLOCH, W. S., and PITTS, W. H. (1959). Physiological evidence that cut optic nerve fibres in the frog regenerate to their proper places in the tectum. *Science* **130**, 1709–10.

McCULLOCH, W. S. and PITTS, W. H. (1943). A logical calculus of the ideas immanent in nervous activity. *Bull. Math. Biophys.* **5**, 115–33.

McINTYRE, A. K., MARK, R. F., and STEINER, J. (1956). Multiple firing at central synapses. *Nature* **178**, 302–4.

MELLON, D. JNR. (1968). *The physiology of sense organs*. Oliver and Boyd, London.

MELZACK, R., KONRAD, K. W., and DUBROVSKY, B. (1969). Prolonged changes in central nervous system activity produced by somatic and reticular stimulation. *Expmtl. Neurol.* **25**, 416–28.

MERRILL, E. G. and WALL, P. D. (1972). Factors forming the edge of a receptive field: the presence of relatively ineffective afferent terminals. *J. Physiol.* **226**, 825–46.

MILLER, S. and KONORSKI, J. (1928). Sur une forme particulière des réflexes conditionnels. *C.r. Soc. biol. Paris* **99**, 1155–7.

MILNER, B. and PENFIELD, W. (1955). The effect of hippocampal lesions on recent memory. *Trans. Am. Neurol. Assoc.* **80**, 42–8.

MINER, N. (1956). Integumental specification of sensory fibers in the development of cutaneous local sign. *J. Comp. Neurol.* **105**, 161–70.

MORRELL, F. (1961). Electrophysiological contributions to the neural basis of learning. *Physiol. Rev.* **41**, 443–94.

MORRELL, F., ENGEL, J. P., and BOURIS, W. (1967). The effect of experience on the firing pattern of visual cortical neurons. *Electroenceph. Clin. Neurophysiol.* **23**, 89.

MOUNTCASTLE, V. B. (1957). Modality and topographic properties of single neurons in the cat's sensory cortex, *J. Neurophysiol.* **20**, 408–34.

MUELLER, R. A., THOENEN, H., and AXELROD, J. (1969). Increase in tyrosine hydroxylase activity after reserpine administration. *J. Pharm. Exp. Ther.* **169**, 74–9.

MURRAY, J. G. and THOMPSON, J. W. (1957). The occurrence and function of collateral sprouting in the sympathetic nervous system of the cat. *J. Physiol.* **135**, 133–62.

OLDS, J. (1972). Learning and the hippocampus. *Rev. Can. Biol.* **31**: *Suppl. printemps*, 215–38.

OLDS, J., DISTERHOFT, J. F., SEGAL, M., KORNBLITH, C. L., and HIRSH, R. (1972). Learning centers of rat brain mapped by measuring latencies of conditioned unit responses. *J. Neurophysiol.* **35**, 202–19.

OLDS, J. and HIRANO, T. (1969). Conditioned responses of hippocampal and other neurons. *Electroenceph. Clin. Neurophysiol.* **26**, 144–58.

PATON, W. D. M. and VIZI, E. S. (1963). The inhibitory action of noradrenaline and adrenaline on acetylcholine output by guinea pig ileum longitudinal muscle strip. *Brit. J. Pharmacol.* **35**, 10–28.

PAVLOV, I. P. (1906). The scientific investigation of the psychical faculties or processes in the higher animals. *Lancet* (*ii*), 911–15.

PHILLIP, J. (1965). Recent thoughts on strabismic amblyopia. *Surgery* **20**, 316–20.

POTTER, L. J. (1969). Synthesis, storage and release of ^{14}C-acetylcholine in isolated rat diaphragm muscles. *J. Physiol.* **206**, 145–66.

PRESTIGE, M. C. (1970). Differentiation degeneration and the role of the periphery: quantitative considerations. In *The neurosciences, second studies program* (ed. F. O. Schmitt), pp. 73–82. Rockefeller University Press, New York.

QUARTERMAIN, D., McEWEN, B. J., and AZMITIA, E. C. JUN. (1972). Recovery of memory following amnesia in the rat and mouse. *J. Comp. Physiol. Psychol.* **79**, 360–70.

RACE, J. JUN (1961). Thyroid hormone control of development of lateral motor column cells in the lumbosacral cord in hypophysectomized *Rana pipiens. Gen. comp. Endocr.* **1**, 322–31.

RAISMAN, G. (1969). Neuronal plasticity in the septal nuclei of the adult rat. *Brain Res.* **14**, 25–48.

RANG, H. P. and RITCHIE, J. M. (1968). On the electrogenic sodium pump in mammalian non-myelinated nerve fibres and its activation by various external cations. *J. Physiol.* **196**, 183–221.

REINIS, S. (1965). The formation of conditioned reflexes in rats after parenteral administration of brain homogenate. *Activ. Nerv. Super.* **7**, 167–8.

RITCHIE, J. M. and STRAUB, R. W. (1957). The hyperpolarization which follows activity in mammalian, non-myelinated fibres. *J. Physiol.* **136**, 80–97.

ROBERTS, R. B. and FLEXNER, L. B. (1969). The biochemical basis of long-term memory. *Quart. Rev. Biophys.* **2**, 135–73.

ROGERS, L. J. and MARK, R. F. (1973). Learning without memory and memory without learning. *Proc. Austral. Physiol. pharm. Soc.* (in the press).

ROSENZWEIG, M. R., BENNETT, E. L., and DIAMOND, M. C. (1972). Chemical and anatomical plasticity of brain: replications and extensions, 1970. In *Macromolecules and behaviour* (ed. J. Gaito). Appleton-Century-Crofts, New York.

ROSENZWEIG, M. R., MOLLGAARD, K., DIAMOND, M. C., and BENNETT, E. C. (1972). Negative as well as positive synaptic changes may store memory, *Psychol. Rev.* **79**, 93–6.

RUSSELL, W. R. and NATHAN, P. W. (1946). Traumatic amnesia. *Brain* **69**, 280–300.

SAHOTA, T. S. and EDWARDS, J. S. (1969). Development of grafted supernumerary legs in the house cricket. *Acheta domesticus. J. Insect Physiol.* **15**, 1367–73.

SAUNDERS, J. C., BOCK, G. R., JAMES, R., and CHEN, C. S. (1972). Effects of priming for audiogenic seizure on auditory evoked responses in the cochlear nucleus and inferior colliculus of BALB/c mice. *Expmtl. Neurol.* **37**, 388–94.

SHOLL, D. A. (1956). *The organization of the cerebral cortex.* Methuen, London.

SKINNER, B. F. (1961). A case history in scientific method. In *Cumulative record*, p. 76–100. Methuen, London.

SLUKIN, W. (1965). *Imprinting and early learning.* Aldine, Chicago.

SOURKES, T. L. (1967). *Nobel prize winners in medicine and physiology*, 1901–65. Abelard-Schuman, London.

SPENCER, W. A. and APRIL, R. S. (1970). Plastic properties of monosynaptic pathways in mammals. In *Short-term changes in neural activity and behaviour* (eds. G. Horn and R. A. Hinde), pp. 433–74. Cambridge University Press.

SPERRY, R. W. (1943a). Effect of 180 degree rotation of the retinal field on visuomotor coordination. *J. Expmtl. Zool.* **92**, 263–79.

SPERRY, R. W. (1943b). Visuomotor coordination in the newt *Triturus vividescens* after regeneration of the optic nerve. *J. Comp. Neurol.* **79**, 33–55.

SPERRY, R. W. (1945). Centripetal regeneration of the 8th cranial nerve root with systematic restoration of vestibular reflexes. *Am. J. Physiol.* **144**, 735–41.

SPERRY, R. W. (1948). Orderly patterning of synaptic associations in regeneration of intracentral fiber tracts mediating visuomotor coordination. *Anat. Res.* **102**, 63–77.

SPERRY, R. W. (1962). Problems of moledular coding. In *Macromolecular specificity and biological memory* (ed. F. O. Schmitt), pp. 70–3. The M.I.T Press, Cambridge, Massachusetts.

SPERRY, R. W. (1963). Chemoaffinity in the orderly growth of nerve fiber patterns and connections. *Proc. Natn. Acad. Sci. U.S.A.* **50**, 703–10.

SPERRY, R. W. and ARORA, H. L. (1963). Color discrimination after optic nerve regeneration in the fish *Astronotus ocellatus. Develop. Biol.* **7**, 234–43.

SPINELLI, D. N., HIRSCH, H. V. B., PHELPS, R. W., and METZLER, J. (1972).

Visual experience as a determinant of the response characteristics of cortical receptive fields in cats. *Expmtl. Brain Res.* **15**, 289–304.

STEWART, W. (1972). Comments on the chemistry of scotophobin. *Nature* **238**, 202–9.

STIRLING, R. V. (1973). The effect of increasing the innervation field sizes of nerves on their reflex response times in salamanders. *J. Physiol.* **229**, 657–79.

STONE, L. S. (1944). Functional polarization in retinal development and its re-establishment in regenerating retinae of rotated grafted eyes. *Proc. Soc. Expmtl. Biol. Med.* **57**, 13–14.

STRUMWASSER, F. (1964). The demonstration and manipulation of a circadian rhythm in a single neuron. In *Circadian clocks* (ed. J. Aschoff), pp. 442–62, North-Holland Publishing Co., Amsterdam.

STRUMWASSER, F. (1967). Types of information stored in single neurons. In *Invertebrate nervous system* (ed. C. A. G. Wiersma), pp. 291–319. University of Chicago Press, Chicago.

SUTTON, T. J. and MARK, R. F. (1973). A study of competitive innervation of hindlimb muscles in *Ambystoma mexicanum*. In preparation.

SZEKELY, G. (1954*a*). Zur Ausbildung der lokalen funktionellen spezifitat der Retina. *Acta. Biol. Acad. Sci. Hung.* **5**, 157–67.

SZEKELY, G. (1954*b*). Untersuchung der Entwicklung optischer Reflexmechanismen an Amphibienlarven. *Acta. Physiol. Acad. Sci. Hung.* **6**, *Suppl.* 18.

SZENTAGOTHAI, J. (1967). The anatomy of complex integrative units in the nervous system. In *Recent development in neurobiology in Hungary* (ed. K. Lissak), vol. 1, pp. 9–45. Akademiai Kiadó, Budapest.

SZILARD, L. (1964). On memory and recall. *Proc. Nat. Acad. Sci. U.S.A.* **51**, 1092–9.

THESLEFF, S. (1960). Supersensitivity of skeletal muscle produced by botulinum toxin. *J. Physiol.* **151**, 598–607.

THOMPSON, R. F. and SPENCER, W. A. (1966). Habituation: a model phenomenon for the study of neuronal substrates of behaviour. *Psychol. Rev.* **173**, 16–43.

THORNDIKE, E. C. (1911). *Animal intelligence*, Hafner, New York.

THORPE, W. H. (1963). *Learning and instinct in animals* (2nd edn.). Methuen, London.

UNGAR, G. (1970). *Molecular mechanisms in memory and learning*. Plenum Press, New York.

UNGAR, G., DESIDERIO, D. M., and PARR, W. (1972). Isolation, identification and synthesis of a specific-behaviour-inducing brain peptide. *Nature* **238**, 198–202.

UNGAR, G. and OCEGUERA-NAVARRO, C. (1965). Transfer of habituation by material extracted from brain. *Nature* **207**, 301–2.

UTTLEY, A. M. (1970). The informon: a network for adaptive pattern recognition. *J. Theor. Biol.* **27**, 31–67.

VOWLES, D. M. (1965). Maze learning and visual discrimination in the wood ant (*Formica rufa*). *Brit. J. Psychol.* **56**, 15–31.

WALL, P. D. and EGGER, M. D. (1971). Formation of new connexions in adult rat brains after partial deafferentation. *Nature* **232**, 542–5.

WALL, P. D. and TAUB, A. (1962). Four aspects of the trigeminal nucleus and a paradox. *J. Neurophysiol.* **25**, 110–26.

WALSH, R. N., BUDTZ-OLSEN, O. E., PENNY, J. E., and CUMMINS, R. A. (1969). The effects of environmental complexity on the histology of the rat hippocampus. *J. comp. Neurol.* **137**, 361–5.

WATSON, J. D. (1970). Molecular biology of the gene (2nd edn.), p. 292. W. A. Benjamin, Menlo Park, California.

WATTS, M. E. and MARK, R. F. (1971). Drug inhibition of memory formation in chickens. II. Short-term memory. *Proc. Roy. Soc. B* **178**, 455–64.

WEILER, I. J. (1966). Restoration of visual acuity after optic nerve section and regeneration in *Astronotus ocellatus*. *Expmtl. Neurol.* **15**, 377–86.

WEISS, P. (1926). The relations between central and peripheral co-ordination. *J. Comp. Neurol.* **40**, 241–51.

WEISS, P. (1931). Selectivity controlling the central–peripheral relations in the nervous system. *Biol. Rev.* **11**, 494–531.

WEISS, P. (1950). Central versus peripheral factors in the development of coordination. *Proc. Assoc. Res. nerve ment. Dis.* **30**, 3–23.

WESTERMAN, R. A. (1965). Specificity in regeneration of optic and olfactory pathways in teleost fish. In *Studies in physiology* (eds. D. R. Curtis and A. K. McIntyre), pp. 263–269. Springer, Berlin.

WIERSMA, C. A. G. (1947). Giant nerve fibre system of the crayfish; a contribution to comparative physiology of synapse. *J. Neurophysiol.* **10**, 23–38.

WIESEL, T. N. and HUBEL, D. H. (1963). Single cell responses in striate cortex of kittens deprived of vision in one eye. *J. Neurophysiol.* **26**, 1003–17.

WIESEL, T. N. and HUBEL, D. H. (1965a). Comparison of the effects of unilateral and bilateral eye closure on cortical unit responses in kittens. *J. Neurophysiol.* **28**, 1029–40.

WIESEL, T. N. and HUBEL, D. H. (1965b). Extent of recovery from the effects of visual deprivation in kittens. *J. Neurophysiol.* **28**, 1060–72.

WICKELGREN, B. (1967). Habituation of spinal motoneurones, *J. Neurophysiol.* **30**, 1404–23.

WOLPERT, L. (1969). Positional information and the spatial pattern of cellular differentiation. *J. Theoret. Biol.* **25**, 1–47.

YOON, M. (1971). Reorganization of retinotectal projection following surgical operations on the optic tectum in goldfish. *Expmtl. Neurol.* **33**, 395–411.

YOON, M. (1972). Reversibility of the reorganization of retinotectal projection in goldfish. *Expmtl. Neurol.* **35**, 565–77.

YOUNG, J. Z. (1964). *A model of the brain.* Clarendon Press, Oxford.

YOUNG, J. Z. (1965). The organization of a memory system. *The Croonian Lecture, Proc. Roy. Soc. B.* **163**, 285–320.

YOUNG, J. Z. (1966). *The memory system of the brain.* Oxford University Press, Oxford.

ZUCKER, R. S. (1972). Crayfish escape behaviour and central synapses. I, II, and III. *J. Neurophysiol.* **35**, 599–651.

Author Index

Subject Index